FECAL INCONTINENCE - CAUSES, MANAGEMENT AND OUTCOME

Edited by **Anthony G. Catto-Smith**

Fecal Incontinence - Causes, Management and Outcome

http://dx.doi.org/10.5772/57038

Edited by Anthony G. Catto-Smith

Contributors

Anthony G. Catto-Smith, Carolyn Coffey, Claudia Regina De Souza Santos, Tania das Graças de Souza Lima, Fernanda Mateus Queiroz Schmidt, Vera Lúcia Conceição de Gouveia Santos, Vittorio Piloni, Roberto Ghiselli, John Camilleri-Brennan, Małgorzata Kołodziejczak, Iwona Sudoł-Szopińska, Misel Trajanovska, Russell Taylor, Abdel Karim Mohamad El Hemaly, Constantine Spanos, Arzu Ilce, Talal A Al-Malki

Published by InTech

Janeza Trdine 9, 51000 Rijeka, Croatia

Publishing Process Manager Iva Lipovic

Technical Editor InTech DTP team

Cover InTech Design team

First published April, 2014

Printed in Croatia

Additional hard copies can be obtained from orders@intechopen.com

Fecal Incontinence - Causes, Management and Outcome, Edited by Anthony G. Catto-Smith

p. cm.

ISBN 978-953-51-1241-9

For EU product safety concerns:
IN TECH d.o.o., Prolaz Marije Krucifikse Kozulić 3, 51000 Rijeka, Croatia,
info@intechopen.com or visit our website at intechopen.com.

Meet the editor

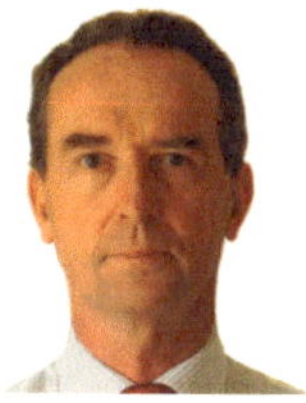

Professor Catto-Smith is Director of the Department of Gastroenterology and Clinical Nutrition at The Royal Children's Hospital, Melbourne. He qualified in medicine from St Bartholomew's Hospital in London, trained in pediatrics in the UK and Australia, then in pediatric gastroenterology at the University of Calgary in Canada. After returning to Melbourne in 1990, he pioneered the introduction of clinical techniques for the measurement of gastrointestinal motility at RCH. He has continued a strong clinical interest in disorders of colorectal function and published extensively in this area. Current research focuses on novel treatment approaches to constipation and fecal incontinence. Other clinical and research interests include the pathogenesis and treatment of Crohn's and Ulcerative Colitis. He is the author of over 140 journal articles.

Contents

Preface

"A good reliable set of bowels is worth more to a man than any quantity of brains" [Josh Billings]

The normal functioning of the gastrointestinal tract is one of the most pivotal yet under-appreciated aspects of good health. Often it is only when something goes wrong that we begin to glimpse the importance of what goes into being well. This is only too true of normal bowel function. The effective and safe management of human waste has been a critical pillar for the development of much of what we have in society today. Once huge mortalities associated with cholera or infantile gastroenteritis are largely forgotten in most western societies. At an individual level, the control of fecal continence is seen as a crucial developmental step in human maturation, with enormous ramifications for self-esteem if it is either not achieved or lost.

Although control of fecal continence superficially appears to be a relatively simple concept, it is surprisingly complex and can be extraordinarily difficult to manage. This book addresses the causes, evaluation, management and outcome for continence of a number of different conditions. The individual authors come with a rich variety of experiences.

The normal acquisition of bowel control in childhood is seen as a crucial developmental step and there is enormous pressure on families whose child is identified as being "slow". This is usually related to variations in physiological development, but can be secondary to anatomical abnormalities such as after the repair of congenital anorectal malformations. It is very difficult to achieve normal physiological functioning with surgery.

A second very important cause of fecal incontinence is that of childbirth-induced traumatic injuries to the pelvic floor with subsequent long-term loss of bowel control. This continues to be an important health issue in the developing world and is covered in the book.

Before proceeding to any effective treatment, it is crucial to understand normal functioning and to be able to meaningfully evaluate the pathophysiology.

The range of different treatment options that are potentially available can be extremely confusing. They include physiological retraining techniques, injectables to supplement sphincter function, and surgery. Defining the correct initial approach can be challenging, but it can be even more difficult to define the next line of management for treatment failures. Many practitioners simply cross their fingers, hoping that it will improve in time.

Good quality clinical research in this area is also surprisingly sparse. Whether it is in defining normal maturation, the advantages or limitations of investigations, or critical evaluation of treatment options, this is clearly an important area to encourage. This book goes some way toward defining future directions for research.

Anthony G. Catto-Smith
Department of Gastroenterology and Clinical Nutrition, Royal Children's Hospital
Professorial Fellow, Department of Paediatrics, University of Melbourne, Australia

Section 1

Pathophysiology

Chapter 1

Childhood Encopresis — Pathophysiology, Evaluation and Treatment

C. Coffey and A.G. Catto-Smith

Additional information is available at the end of the chapter

http://dx.doi.org/10.5772/57071

1. Introduction

Encopresis is defined as persistent faecal incontinence without associated anatomic abnormality. It is a common, disabling condition of children often associated with functional defaecation disorders potentially open to nonsurgical treatments. It is considered to be primarily a disorder associated with chronic constipation, with stool retention in 96% of children over the age of four years presenting with faecal incontinence. [1]

The symptom of constipation is defined broadly as difficulty or delay in defaecation [2], often associated with large calibre stools and the presence of stool in the rectal ampulla. [3-5] Anecdotal evidence from parents often shows a transition from early simple constipation to chronic constipation, faecal retention and soiling. [6]

Constipation may not be easy to identify on history. Barr et al. noted that 45 percent of children when asked the most commonly used screening question for constipation relating to frequency of bowel motions gave an answer within the normal range. [5] These children were obviously constipated based on other criteria. Some children with encopresis have daily bowel motions but apparently incomplete evacuation as evidenced by periodic passage of very large amounts of stool. [7] Conversely, infrequent defaecation alone may not indicate constipation as this may simply represent the lower limit of normality. [8] In the literature the terms 'constipation' and 'faecal retention' are used interchangeably.

A period of continence is often defined as a period of at least one month without faecal incontinence. However, the frequency of soiling episodes does not necessarily correlate with severity of constipation. [9] Soiling in childhood encopresis is variable in quantity and frequency and may occur in the range of monthly to many times a day. It can occur at night but rarely exclusively so. [10] Children may have always soiled (primary) or may have commenced soiling after a period of continence (secondary) with a third to half of children presenting with primary encopresis. [11, 12]

The underlying pathologies resulting in childhood faecal retention remain relatively poorly understood. Colonic motility, large gut innervation, cyclic anal activity, bowel sensation and evacuation release, as well as behavioural factors may all contribute in varying degrees to the condition known generically as constipation with secondary encopresis. Encopresis involving soiling without evidence of stool accumulation and in the absence of any obvious anatomic abnormality does occur but there are no studies which have specifically and usefully examined functional disorders in this group.

Some authors attribute soiling and the generally associated faecal retention solely or predominantly to psychogenic causes. Halpern [13] reviewed the child rearing practices and personality types said to precipitate encopresis, but pointed to the lack of firm evidence associating inadequate parenting with soiling. Children with encopresis have been found to have a higher incidence of maladjustment than the normal population, but this is far from universal and more importantly has been observed to improve with symptomatic remission. [11, 14-16] It is likely therefore that the symptom of encopresis is at least contributing to the behaviour problems rather than the reverse. The stress on the child, his/her family, friends and teachers resulting from prolonged faecal incontinence is obvious but it should not distract from the need to identify and correct any functional abnormality that may exist. [16]

2. Epidemiology and natural history

Boys are far more prone to encopresis than girls, with the prevalence of encopresis amongst 7 to 8 year old boys 2.3 percent and amongst girls of 0.7 percent in the classic study from Stockholm. [17] The Isle of Wight survey found that 1.3 percent of 11 year old boys and 0.3 percent of girls were incontinent of stool [18], and similar data has recently been reported from the Netherlands. [19]

Approximately 70 to 80% of children presenting with encopresis are boys. [10, 11, 20, 21] The proportion of boys in studies of children with chronic constipation is approximately 60 percent. [3, 22-24]

In adults the picture is reversed with women being more inclined to suffer from constipation8, [25] and incontinence. [26, 27] However, in the clinical group of 276 patients described by Speakman and Henry, if men and women who had had previous surgery or trauma and the women who had a history of difficult vaginal delivery were discounted then the remaining patients consisted of 6 women and 4 men. Obviously when comparing childhood and adult prevalence of any disorder it is necessary to discount adult conditions for which there is no paediatric equivalent.

Faecal incontinence tends to be underreported in medical histories, [28] likely leading to systematic underestimation of its incidence and prevalence in adults. In one study, only 5% of patients with self-reported faecal incontinence had this recorded in their medical history. [28]

http://dx.doi.org/10.5772/57071

Of the 46% controls who responded to the questionnaire, 5% indicated they experienced faecal soiling. It was suggested that either the doctor might be reluctant to treat the problem, or alternatively that they regarded it as a minor symptom. Therefore assessment of the recovery rate of children with encopresis by comparison of reported prevalences is open to gross inaccuracies. It seems likely that the same bias occurs in paediatric reporting. In their study of 176 consecutively referred children with constipation, Arhan et al. [29] reported a referral diagnosis of encopresis in 8% but in fact 68% of the 176 children suffered from this symptom.

There are functional differences in continence mechanisms between normal adult men and women. These include greater activity of both sphincters in men and a lower rectal volume to reach the threshold for desire to defaecate in women. [30-32] There are dangers inherent in extrapolation from the physiology of adults to children but it has suggested that gender differences also exist in paediatric anorectal function which might explain the greater proportion of boys with anorectal dysfunction. To date most studies which have included a comparison group of control children have not found evidence to support this suggestion. Corazziari did study 78 healthy children as a comparison group for 63 chronically constipated children and found no gender difference in stool frequency or total gastrointestinal transit time. [24] Only 25 (13 boys) children had manometric studies and there were no gender differences identified. Similarly, Meunier et al. found no significant gender differences in two control groups of normal children (n= 32 and 31). [23, 33]

3. Physiology of normal continence and defaecation

In order to investigate continence and defaecation disorders it is first necessary to understand these processes in a normal person. Unfortunately the literature only provides detailed studies of normal adults and so we are in the position of having to extrapolate these findings to children.

Stool frequency in Western communities decreases in the first years of life and then appears to plateau, but there is some evidence that this is not the case in developing communities for which there are no significant age-related differences. [34] Corazziari [24] observed that bowel frequency was significantly higher in children younger than three years than those of 3 to 12 years but found no difference in total gastrointestinal transit time. Normal frequency in the older age group was considered to be between 4 and 9 bowel actions per week. In young adults 5 to 12 bowel actions per week can be considered to be normal with males defaecating significantly more frequently than females. [35]

Continence is maintained by the physical resistance to the passage of faeces moving from the rectosigmoid into the rectum and thence through the anal canal. [36] Stool transfer into the rectum usually occurs as a result of colonic high-amplitude propagated contractions, which are more likely to occur after wakening and meals. The rectum is generally collapsed before the arrival of faeces, which then result in distension, rectal contraction, a sensation of urgency, reflex relaxation of the internal anal sphincter and semi-voluntary relaxations of pelvic floor muscles. If defaecation does not occur, rectal contractions and the sense of urgency slowly subside with the rectum accommodating to continuing distension. Resistance to the movement of stool into the rectum allows its accumulation in the distal colon.

The movement of faeces into the distal rectum from the sigmoid colon is impeded by its two lateral angulations and its spiral folds. [37] Resistance to movement through the anorectum is provided by the sharp anteroposterior angulation and the anal sphincters. The anorectal angle is maintained by the striated pelvic muscles, mainly the puborectalis. The anal sphincters form a high pressure zone consisting of two overlapping muscles: the internal anal sphincter (IAS) composed of smooth muscle, and the external anal sphincter (EAS) composed of striated muscle. Tonic change in the IAS is entirely reflex whilst that in the EAS is under voluntary control. Contraction of the puborectalis sling in conjunction with contraction of the EAS is thought to assist the role of this sphincter. It does not appear to play as important a role in the maintenance of continence as the EAS.

The two sphincters can function independently of each other, depending on the need to accommodate faecal matter, ascertain the nature of the rectal contents, preserve continence or to defaecate. At rest the sphincters maintain a high pressure zone which has an asymmetric profile with the highest pressures in the outermost sphincter area. [37] The asymmetry is largely maintained by contraction of the EAS which predominantly surrounds the distal anal canal and is submaximally tonically active under resting conditions. However, approximately 80 percent of the total sphincter tone is due to the activity of the IAS. Cyclical variations in resting pressure within the anal canal including spontaneous relaxations of the sphincter have been observed in adults [32, 38] and in children. [39] There is a reduction in IAS tone, resting EAS activity and colonic motor activity during sleep in adults. [37] There is some suggestion that the EAS undergoes periodic change in tonic activity. [40]

With the arrival of sufficient faeces in the rectal canal to cause it to distend to a threshold volume there is a reflex relaxation of the IAS accompanied by contraction of the EAS. This rectoanal inhibitory reflex (RAIR) is associated with an increase in rectal pressure due to rectal contraction and within one second a transient sensation. [41] The triggering of the RAIR appears to be dependent on the rate of rectal distension: slow continuous filling allows a greater volume to collect before the IAS relaxes. Further increases in rectal contents beyond this threshold produce a gradation of sensation from that of wind, to an urge to defaecate, to the experience of pain. [42] Following each increase in rectal contents and volume, the EAS recovers resting tone after the brief increase in activity. There is however a rebound increase in resting pressure of the IAS and the baseline rectal pressure increases for a period accompanied by an increase in rectal contractions. [30]

The rectal contractions reduce earlier with slower rates of filling but accommodation of the rectal contents can occur longitudinally without the necessity of relaxation of the rectal wall. [43] The increases in rectal contractions and axial pressures possibly tamp the stool into the proximal anal canal thereby increasing the defaecatory urge. [44] As the volume increases the relaxation of the IAS increases in strength and duration until recovery no longer occurs and there is a sustained relaxation. Parallel to this the contraction of the EAS increases in strength and duration, maintaining continence. Prior to sustained relaxation of the IAS during the resting phases, Frenckner [45] determined that the IAS is responsible for just over half the anal tone and is therefore still important in maintaining continence.

The progression from mild to acute urgency generally occurs with the attainment of sustained increase in rectal tone and dilatation of the IAS. The sense of urgency is likely due to activation of stretch receptors in the proximal rectum or sigmoid colon. [43] There is disagreement about whether acute urgency and sustained relaxation of the IAS always occur together in normal children [4, 16, 46] while in adults Sun et al. [43] found no evidence for this.

There are significant differences between age groups in normal children in both the maximal tolerable rectal volume, and the threshold volume required to elicit rectal contractions (rectorectal reflex). [33] The thresholds for these increased and decreased respectively with increasing age.

Although some component of the EAS response to the inhibitory reflex is spinal (as it is observed to an extent in paraplegic patients) [47] depending on the level of the lesion it is susceptible to conscious control and therefore must be modulated by CNS involvement. [48] During sleep there is no diminution of the IAS response but there is a significant reduction in the EAS component.

Very high levels of rectal distension can be associated with reflex abolition of both EAS and IAS activity causing a profound reduction in anal pressure [41] resulting in automatic defaecation. [49] This has been noted in normal children [4, 50] and adults. [51] This reflex is present in paraplegic patients with intact peripheral nerves and distal spinal reflexes so it is probably autonomous. [47]

The sensory receptors are complex in that not only the presence but also the nature of rectal contents are perceived, and the sensation due to IAS relaxation is felt differently from that due to rectal distension. [52] Receptors exist in the anal canal and may exist in the rectum and the muscles of the pelvic floor. There is disagreement about the origins of rectal sensation, whether mediated by receptors in the pelvic floor and not in the rectum, or whether as Sun [43] and Loening-Baucke [53] have postulated there are at least two types of rectal receptors: rapidly adapting mucosal receptors and slowly adapting mechanoreceptors in or on the rectal wall, as well as the possibility of some in the sigmoid colon.

Sun [41] found that the duration of IAS relaxation and sensation in adults were not correlated although the former was always shorter than the latter. However, a strong association was found between the durations of EAS contraction and sensation. Transient sensation was not generally perceived if rectal contractions were not elicited and the EAS did not contract unless perception occurred. [30] Buser et al. [52] found that some adults with faecal incontinence did experience sensation at a time when EAS contraction was absent, so postulated that the EAS contracts as the result of rather than the cause of sensation. Read and Read [54] have suggested that the role of anal sensation receptors, as opposed to the rectal complex, may not be to preserve continence but to identify the rectal contents or signal the end of defaecation. [49] If this is the case then the RAIR allows testing of the rectal contents by these receptors, providing conscious information on which suitable actions may be taken. It has been suggested the spontaneous cyclical IAS relaxations fulfil the same purpose. [38]

An alternative or supplementary mechanism for the identification of the physical nature of faeces may be associated with the different rates of distension of the rectal wall accompanying the propulsion of material from the distal colon. As well as differences in RAIR thresholds, rapid rectal distension has been found to produce a different sensation from gradual distension to the same volume so that distinction between these may provide the discriminatory information. [43] However, whatever the order and origins of stimuli, it is obvious that once the rectal contents have reached the threshold for reflex relaxation of the IAS then at least subconscious awareness of stool in the rectum and immediate contraction of the EAS are essential for the preservation of continence. The ability to experience a sense of urgency before profound reflex anal dilatation occurs is likewise essential.

With an increase in intra-abdominal pressure there is a reflex compensatory increase in EAS activity to a level which provides an anal pressure in excess of the rectal pressure. [30] This allows continence to be maintained when coughing, sneezing, blowing up balloons, laughing or any other activity which poses a threat by its effect on abdominal pressure. Voluntary squeezing or tightening up of the EAS to maintain continence involves no increase in intra-abdominal pressure. [6]

Voluntary defaecation takes place in three phases. Initially there is an increase in abdominal pressure and rectal pressure brought about by closure of the glottis, fixation of the diaphragm and contraction of abdominal, perianal and hamstring muscles combined with contraction of the puborectalis sling and both sphincters. [37] Then the pelvic muscles relax allowing straightening of the rectoanal angle and of both sphincters. The normal anorectal angle at rest is approximately 90° and increases to 125° during straining. At the same time strong colorectal contractions assist expulsion of the stool and the anal sphincters relax. Electrical activity in the EAS is greatly reduced at this stage. Schuster [49] suggested that this relaxation takes place when the threshold for automatic defaecation is reached. As defaecation proceeds the rectal pressure gradually falls. The third stage involves the return to the original state after a rebound contraction of the anal sphincters.

It can be seen from the complex nature of continence and defaecation that there are many opportunities for problems to occur both through physiological deficits and disordered processes. [36] Insufficient IAS or EAS resting tone, inadequate or delayed EAS response to the rectoanal inhibitory reflex, elevated or absent threshold of sensation from rectal distension and a blunted feeling of urgency have all been proposed as possible causes or at least contributors to faecal incontinence. Inadequate colonic propulsion, failure of the IAS to relax, inappropriate contraction of the EAS and puborectalis, failure of the levators to lift the pelvic floor, luminal obstruction or an impairment in the central control of defaecation may singly or in combination result in obstructed defaecation. Failure to relax the striated musculature of the pelvic floor during straining has been termed anismus [55] and probably results in incomplete evacuation, faecal retention, chronic distension of the rectum, and possibly concomitant reduction in sensation leading to soiling or, at least, to its continuation. [56] Attempts to identify pathophysiology which may be present in children with faecal incontinence have largely concentrated on studies of resting anorectal pressure and motility characteristics, sensation, the RAIR and the investigation of anismus.

4. Treatment

The aim of treatment is to for the patient to achieve the ability to be in charge of his/her own continence and defaecation. [57, 58] To this end the any significant faecal impaction needs to be relieved and a regular output established. Treatment for encopresis falls into three stages with the first being initial disimpaction with commencement of maintenance laxatives or prokinetic agents. The second stage is the establishment of a good bowel habit by the use of behaviour modification; and thirdly, the correction, if necessary, of abnormal defaecation dynamics. The first two modes of treatment are frequently adequate to resolve the problem but if the encopresis is refractory. Many children respond well but there is undoubtedly a group who continue to have long term problems past puberty. [59]

4.1. Laxatives

Laxative treatment regimens vary in detail but generally aim to produce one to two bowel actions per day. The extent of the faecal retention determines the type of medication. Polyethylene glycol ("macrogol") based regimens are increasingly accepted as a first line, but there is still an occasional place for stimulant laxatives such as senna derivatives or bisacodyl. [57] Enemas and suppositories are now only infrequently used for disimpaction. Increased fibre is of use only if the current intake is inadequate. [58]

4.2. Behaviour modification

Concurrently with laxative medication, a star chart with a reward system both for successful defaecation in the toilet and for soil-free days can be used as positive reinforcement aimed towards achieving an improvement in toileting habit. Regular sits three times a day for 5-10 minutes with a minimum of distraction is an effective regimen [11] In addition, clarification of the physiology of encopresis to parents and children to alleviate guilt is very important, as is attentive follow-up to maintain compliance and monitor progress. In a referred population of children presenting with encopresis this regimen can be expected to result in complete remission from soiling in approximately half [11, 12, 60] and in addition to be independent of laxatives in the same or less.[4, 9]

4.3. Biofeedback for treatment of anismus

The rationale for the development of biofeedback had been to provide a correction of disturbed anorectal dynamics, and especially for paradoxical sphincteric contraction or anismus. [61] The method recommended for biofeedback generally is the same as, or an adaption of, anorectal manometry with some sort of visual or auditory feedback of sphincteric contraction. Unfortunately critical evaluation in controlled studies has failed to provide evidence of superior efficacy to standard treatments. [62, 63]

5. Discussion

Encopresis in childhood is an important cause of soiling, with socially disabling consequences. It is usually associated with constipation and is thought to be secondary to periodic relaxation of the anal sphincters in the presence of a loaded rectum with secondary seepage. The pathophysiology of disturbed anorectal function is relatively poorly studied in children and results often interpreted with data obtained from adult studies. Most children do have some type of manometric abnormality and many have a degree of rectal enlargement. Dynamic abnormalities also exist and the best studied is paradoxical sphincteric contraction or "anis-mus'.

Treatment regimens which include a combination laxatives for disimpaction and maintenance, together with behavioural interventions centred around encouraging toileting are generally effective but there is a group of children who go on to have significant long term problems.

Author details

C. Coffey[1] and A.G. Catto-Smith[1,2*]

*Address all correspondence to: tony.cattosmith@rch.org.au

1 Dept of Gastroenterology, Royal Children's Hospital Melbourne, Australia

2 Dept of Pediatrics, University of Melbourne, Australia

References

[1] Loening-Baucke V. Biofeedback therapy for fecal incontinence. Dig Dis 1990;8:112-24.

[2] Clayden GS. Constipation and soiling in childhood. Br Med J 1976;1:515-7.

[3] Abrahamian FP, Lloyd-Still JD. Chronic constipation in childhood: a longitudinal study of 186 patients. J Pediatr Gastroenterol Nutr 1984;3:460-7.

[4] Loening-Baucke VA. Sensitivity of the sigmoid colon and rectum in children treated for chronic constipation. J Pediatr Gastroenterol Nutr 1984;3:454-9.

http://dx.doi.org/10.5772/57071

[5] Barr RG, Levine MD, Wilkinson RH, Mulvihill D. Chronic and occult stool retention: a clinical tool for its evaluation in school-aged children. Clin Pediatr (Phila) 1979;18:674, 676, 677-9, passim.

[6] Loening-Baucke V. Modulation of abnormal defecation dynamics by biofeedback treatment in chronically constipated children with encopresis. J Pediatr 1990;116:214-22.

[7] Loening-Baucke V. Encopresis. Curr Opin Pediatr 2002;14:570-575.

[8] Sandler RS, Jordan MC, Shelton BJ. Demographic and dietary determinants of constipation in the US population. Am J Public Health 1990;80:185-9.

[9] Loening-Baucke VA. Factors responsible for persistence of childhood constipation. J Pediatr Gastroenterol Nutr 1987;6:915-22.

[10] Levine MD. Children with encopresis: A descriptive analysis. Pediatrics 1975;56:412-416.

[11] Nolan T, Debelle G, Oberklaid F, Coffey C. Randomised trial of laxatives in treatment of childhood encopresis. Lancet 1991;338:523-527.

[12] Levine MD, Bakow H. Children with encopresis: a study of treatment outcome. Pediatrics 1976;58:845-52.

[13] Halpern WI. The treatment of encopretic children. J Am Acad Child Psychiatry 1977;16:478-99.

[14] Levine MD, Mazonson P, Bakow H. Behavioral symptom substitution in children cured of encopresis. Am J Dis Child 1980;134:663-7.

[15] Gabel S, Hegedus AM, Wald A, Chandra R, Chiponis D. Prevalence of behavior problems and mental health utilization among encopretic children: implications for behavioral pediatrics. J Dev Behav Pediatr 1986;7:293-7.

[16] Clayden GS, Lawson JO. Investigation and management of long-standing chronic constipation in childhood. Arch Dis Child 1976;51:918-23.

[17] Bellman M. Studies on encopresis. Acta Paediatr Scand 1966;170:1-151.

[18] Rutter M, Tizard J, Whitmore K. Education, health, and behaviour; psychological and medical study of childhood development. Wiley, 1970.

[19] van der Wal MF, Benninga MA, Hirasing RA. The prevalence of encopresis in a multicultural population. Journal of Pediatric Gastroenterology & Nutrition 2005;40:345-8.

[20] Loening-Baucke V. Factors determining outcome in children with chronic constipation and faecal soiling. Gut 1989;30:999-1006.

[21] Wald A, Chandra R, Chiponis D, Gabel S. Anorectal function and continence mechanisms in childhood encopresis. J Pediatr Gastroenterol Nutr 1986;5:346-51.

[22] Partin JC, Hamill SK, Fischel JE, Partin JS. Painful defecation and fecal soiling in children. Pediatrics 1992;89:1007-9.

[23] Meunier P, Marechal JM, de Beaujeu MJ. Rectoanal pressures and rectal sensitivity studies in chronic childhood constipation. Gastroenterology 1979;77:330-6.

[24] Corazziari E, Cucchiara S, Staiano A, Romaniello G, Tamburrini O, Torsoli A, Auricchio S. Gastrointestinal transit time, frequency of defecation, and anorectal manometry in healthy and constipated children. J Pediatr 1985;106:379-82.

[25] Loening-Baucke VA, Cruikshank BM. Abnormal defecation dynamics in chronically constipated children with encopresis. J Pediatr 1986;108:562-6.

[26] Emery Y, Descos L, Meunier P, Louis D, Valancogne G, Weil G. [Terminal constipation caused by abdominopelvic asynchrony: analysis of etiological, clinical, manometric data and therapeutic results after rehabilitation by biofeedback]. Gastroenterol Clin Biol 1988;12:6-11.

[27] Speakman CT, Henry MM. The work of an anorectal physiology laboratory. Baillieres Clin Gastroenterol 1992;6:59-73.

[28] Enck P, Bielefeldt K, Rathmann W, Purrmann J, Tschope D, Erckenbrecht JF. Epidemiology of faecal incontinence in selected patient groups. Int J Colorectal Dis 1991;6:143-146.

[29] Arhan P, Devroede G, Jehannin B, Faverdin C, Revillon Y, Lefevre D, Pellerin D. Idiopathic disorders of fecal continence in children. Pediatrics 1983;71:774-9.

[30] Sun WM, Read NW. Anorectal function in normal human subjects: effect of gender. Int J Colorectal Dis 1989;4:188-96.

[31] Rasmussen OO, Colstrup H, Lose G, Christiansen J. A technique for the dynamic assessment of anal sphincter function. Int J Colorectal Dis 1990;5:135-41.

[32] Pedersen IK, Christiansen J. A study of the physiological variation in anal manometry. Br J Surg 1989;76:69-70.

[33] Meunier P, Louis D, Jaubert de Beaujeu M. Physiologic investigation of primary chronic constipation in children: comparison with the barium enema study. Gastroenterology 1984;87:1351-7.

[34] Myo K, Thein Win N, Kyaw-Hla S, Thein Thein M, Bolin TD. A prospective study on defecation frequency, stool weight, and consistency. Arch Dis Child 1994;71:311-3; discussion 313-4.

[35] Sandler RS, Drossman DA. Bowel habits in young adults not seeking health care. Dig Dis Sci 1987;32:841-5.

[36] Bharucha AE. Fecal Incontinence. In: Parkman HP, McCallum RW, Rao SSC, eds. GI Motility Testing. Thorofare, New Jersey: Slack Incorporated, 2011:383-397.

[37] Bharucha AE. Pelvic floor: anatomy and function. Neurogastroenterol Motil 2006;18:507-19.

[38] Enck P, Eggers E, Koletzko S, Erckenbrecht JF. Spontaneous variation of anal "resting" pressure in healthy humans. Am J Physiol 1991;261:G823-6.

[39] Loening-Baucke VA, Younoszai MK. Abnormal and sphincter response in chronically constipated children. J Pediatr 1982;100:213-8.

[40] Kumar D, Williams NS, Waldron D, Wingate DL. Prolonged manometric recording of anorectal motor activity in ambulant human subjects: evidence of periodic activity. Gut 1989;30:1007-11.

[41] Sun WM, Read NW, Miner PB. Relation between rectal sensation and anal function in normal subjects and patients with faecal incontinence. Gut 1990;31:1056-61.

[42] Tantiphlachiva K, Rao SSC. Anorectal Manometry. In: Parkman HP, McCallum RW, Rao SSC, eds. GI Motility. Thorofare, New Jersey: Slack Incorporated, 2011:163-178.

[43] Sun WM, Read NW, Prior A, Daly JA, Cheah SK, Grundy D. Sensory and motor responses to rectal distention vary according to rate and pattern of balloon inflation. Gastroenterology 1990;99:1008-15.

[44] Bharucha AE, Croak AJ, Gebhart JB, Berglund LJ, Seide BM, Zinsmeister AR, An KN, Bharucha AE, Croak AJ, Gebhart JB, Berglund LJ, Seide BM, Zinsmeister AR, An K-N. Comparison of rectoanal axial forces in health and functional defecatory disorders. American Journal of Physiology - Gastrointestinal & Liver Physiology 2006;290:G1164-9.

[45] Frenckner B, Euler CV. Influence of pudendal block on the function of the anal sphincters. Gut 1975;16:482-9.

[46] Molnar D, Taitz LS, Urwin OM, Wales JK. Anorectal manometry results in defecation disorders. Arch Dis Child 1983;58:257-61.

[47] Frenckner B. Function of the anal sphincters in spinal man. Gut 1975;16:638-44.

[48] Whitehead WE, Orr WC, Engel BT, Schuster MM. External anal sphincter response to rectal distention: learned response or reflex. Psychophysiology 1982;19:57-62.

[49] Schuster MM. The riddle of the sphincters. Gastroenterology 1975;69:249-62.

[50] Aaronson I, Nixon HH. A clinical evaluation of anorectal pressure studies in the diagnosis of Hirschsprung's disease. Gut 1972;13:138-46.

[51] Williamson JL, Nelson RL, Orsay C, Pearl RK, Abcarian H. A comparison of simultaneous longitudinal and radial recordings of anal canal pressures. Dis Colon Rectum 1990;33:201-6.

[52] Buser WD, Miner PB, Jr. Delayed rectal sensation with fecal incontinence. Successful treatment using anorectal manometry. Gastroenterology 1986;91:1186-91.

[53] Loening-Baucke V, Read NW, Yamada T. Further evaluation of the afferent nervous pathways from the rectum. Am J Physiol 1992;262:G927-33.

[54] Read MG, Read NW. Role of anorectal sensation in preserving continence. Gut 1982;23:345-7.

[55] Preston DM, Lennard-Jones JE. Anismus in chronic constipation. Dig Dis Sci 1985;30:413-8.

[56] Catto-Smith AG, Nolan TM, Coffey CM. Clinical significance of anismus in encopresis. J Gastroenterol Hepatol 1998;13:955-960.

[57] Catto-Smith A, Chase J, Edgar D, Fields J, Gibb S, Grattan B, Johnston M, Josephs K. Impact Paediatric Bowel Care Pathway: Australia: The Continence Foundation of Australia, 2007.

[58] Catto-Smith AG. 5. Constipation and toileting issues in children. Med J Aust 2005;182:242-6.

[59] van Ginkel R, Reitsma JB, Buller HA, van Wijk MP, Taminiau JA, Benninga MA. Childhood constipation: longitudinal follow-up beyond puberty. Gastroenterology 2003;125:357-63.

[60] Lowery SP, Srour JW, Whitehead WE, Schuster MM. Habit training as treatment of encopresis secondary to chronic constipation. J Pediatr Gastroenterol Nutr 1985;4:397-401.

[61] Rao SS, Enck P, Loening-Baucke V. Biofeedback therapy for defecation disorders. Dig Dis 1997;15 Suppl 1:78-92.

[62] Loening-Baucke V. Biofeedback training in children with functional constipation. A critical review. Dig Dis Sci 1996;41:65-71.

[63] Nolan T, Catto-Smith T, Coffey C, Wells J. Randomised controlled trial of biofeedback training in persistent encopresis with anismus. Arch Dis Child 1998;79:131-135.

Chapter 2

Fecal Incontinence

Arzu Ilce

Additional information is available at the end of the chapter

http://dx.doi.org/10.5772/57502

1. Introduction

Fecal incontinence (FI) is defined as the recurrent, involuntary passing of solid or liquid stool [1-5]. FI is a common condition that results in significant physical and psychological disability [6].

FI includes the inability to hold a bowel movement until reaching a toilet as well as passing stool into one's underwear without being aware of it happening. Feces is solid waste that is passed as a bowel movement and includes undigested food, bacteria, mucus, and dead cells. Mucus is a clear liquid that coats and protects tissues in the digestive system [3]. FI is a challenging condition of diverse etiology and devastating psychosocial impact [1,3,4]. It severely impacts on the quality of life of many sufferers and their families, often being given as the reason for admission to a care home [7]. Therefore FI can be upsetting and embarrassing. Many people with FI feel ashamed and try to hide the problem. However, people with FI should not be afraid or embarrassed to talk with their health care provider. FI is often caused by a medical problem and treatment is available [1].

Although FI can be both emotionally and socially debilitating, the embarrassment associated with it is so great that it often prevents patients from seeking much needed help from their health care providers. Nursing care begins with case finding and continues through conservative management, which has greatly improved over the past 15 years [8].

2. Epidemiology

FI affects approximately 5% of the general population but its prevalence increases with age. Nearly 18 million United States (US) adults, about one in 12, have FI. FI is common in women; 1:1,010 women in the United States have FI. Nearly 70% of patients with FI have never discussed it with a physician. People of any age can have a bowel control problem, though FI is more common in older adults. Approximately 70% of institutionalized older adults have FI. Obstetric injury is the primary reason for FI in women. Forty-three percent of women who undergo anal sphincter repair following birth still experience FI 12 weeks after surgery, and 11% report FI for as long as 18 months after surgery. FI is common among women with pelvic floor disorders; 20% of women affected by urinary incontinence have FI [4,9-11].

3. Risk factors

FI has many causes, including; diarrhea or constipation, muscle damage or weakness, nerve damage or trauma, loss of stretch in the rectum, aging, congenital disorders, hemorrhoids and rectal prolapse, rectocele, inactivity [1,7,12].

Having any of the following can increase the risk: disease or injury that damages the nervous system; poor overall health from multiple chronic, or long lasting, illnesses, a difficult childbirth with injuries to the pelvic floor, the muscles, ligaments and tissues that support the uterus, vagina, bladder, and rectum [9-11]. Apart from these there are many etiologic factors are given in table 1 [8].

Additional risk factors include obesity [4]. More than 50% of US women are overweight (body mass index 25-30 kg/m^2) or obese (body mass index, 30 kg/ m^2), and the prevalence of obesity is increasing by almost 6% per year [6].

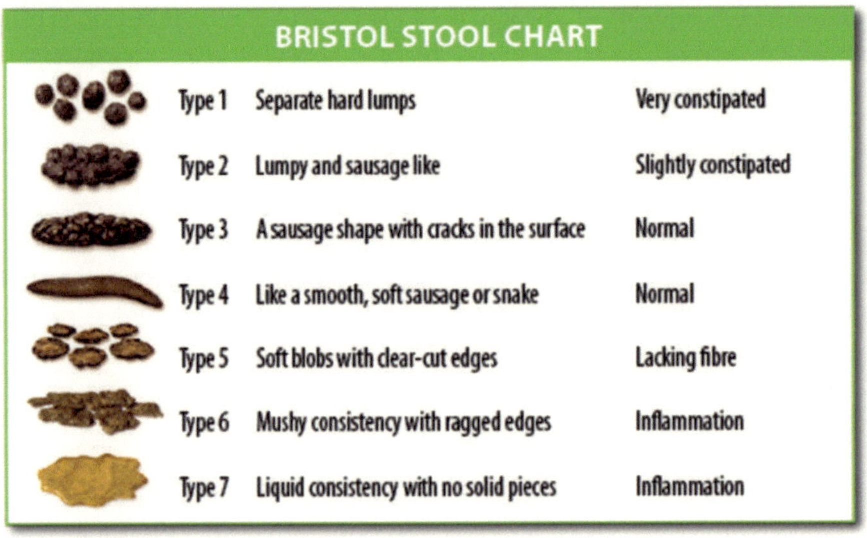

Figure 1. Bristol Stool Chart [13]

http://dx.doi.org/10.5772/57502

Etiologic factors
Perianorectal trauma
Anal sphincter injury
Obstetric procedures or childbirth
Anorectal surgery complications
Pelvic fracture
Abnormal anal sphincter or pelvic floor function
Rectal prolapse
Chronic straining
Neurologic disorders
Spinal cord
Brain injuries, stroke and cerebrovascular disease
Myelomeningocele
Multiple sclerosis
Neuropathy (as may occur in diabetes, for example)
Loose stool consistency or bowel irritation or inflammation
Diarrhea
Gastrointestinal infections
Inflammatory bowel disease or irritable bowel syndrome
Short bowel syndrome resulting from bowel resection
Radiation enteritis
Obstruction and overflow
Impaction
Neoplasms
Medications with antimotility adverse effects
Cognitive or functional disability
Dementia or delirium
Decreased mobility (resulting from stroke, arthritis, lower back problems, or weakness)
Restraints
Inability to access the toilet independently for any reason
Congenital anorectal malformations
Imperforate anus
Hirschsprung's disease
İdiopathic incontinence

Table 1. Etiologic factors of FI [8]

The ideal stool consistency is type three or four on the Bristol stool chart (figure 1). Type one and two stools are hard and can be difficult to pass. Type five, six and seven stools are soft to liquid hard to retain and make it difficult for the person with FI to remain continent [12].

Some medication can cause constipation or diarrhea such as pain medications, iron and depression (table 2) [12].

Medications that cause constipation	
Medication group	Example
Opiates	Morphine sulphate
Codeine based analgesia	Co-dydramol, co-codamol
Iron preparations	Ferrous sulphate
Anticholinergics	Oxybutinin
Diureties	Frusemide
Antidepressants	Amitriptyline, citalopram
Antispasmodics	Propantheline
Antihypertensives	Captopril
Antipsychotics	Risperidone
Medications that cause diarrhea	
Medication group	Example
Digitals	Digoxin
Antidepressants	Fluoxetine (Prozac)
Antidiabetics	Metformin
Antiobesity	Orlistat

Table 2. Medications that cause constipation and diarrhea [12].

Additionally, antibiotics can affect the bacreria in the gut which can increase the risk of developing *Clostridium difficile* and other forms of diarrhea [12].

4. Assesment/ Diagnosis

Health care providers diagnose FI based on a person's lifestyl, medical history, physical exam, and medical test results [2,12,14].

A stool diary is a chart for recording daily bowel movement details. Medical history enables the assessor to work out the possible causes or contributing factors that have led to the

http://dx.doi.org/10.5772/57502

development of FI. Some of these factors can be easily treated. while others may require management.

The healthcare professional should check the condition of the anorectal skin. Enzymes present in faeces can cause incontinence dermatitis, especially if the person has also incontinence of urine. Older people who are living in nursing homes have an increased risk of developing incontinence dermatitis, because large number of residents have continance problems. The healthcare professional should check the anal region for abnormalities such as external haemorroids, skin tags, rectal prolapse, and an anus that gapes open. A cognitive assessment is essential when assessing the older person who has FI. When staff are fully aware of any problems wiih memory and reasonlng, they can devise a plan to treat or manage incontinance [2,12,14].

The person may be referred to a doctor who specializes in problems of the digestive system, such as a gastroenterologist, proctologist, or colorectal surgeon, or a doctor who specializes in problems of the urinary and reproductive systems, such as a urologist or urogynecologist. The specialist will perform a physical exam and may suggest one or more of the following medical tests: Anal manometry, anal ultrasound, magnetic resonance imaging (MRI), defecography, flexible sigmoidoscopy or colonoscopy, anal electromyography (EMG) [2,12,14].

5. Treatment

Fecal incontinence is not a disease but a symptom and can be treate. Treatment for FI may include one or more of the following: eating, diet, and nutrition, medications, bowel training, pelvic floor exercises and biofeedback, surgery, rectal irrigation, colostomy [11,14].

Eating, Diet, and Nutrition: A food diary should list foods eaten, portion size, and when FI occurs. After a few days, the diary may show a link between certain foods and FI. A food diary can also be helpful to a health care provider treating a person with FI [1,9,15].

Dietary modifications are often included as an early treatment strategy for FI, but minimal data exist to guide the recommendations on types of dietary changes. Increasing soluble fiber intake has been shown to improve FI. Overweight and obese women report a high prevalence of monthly FI associated with low dietary fiber intake. Increasing dietary fiber may be a treatment for FI [6]. If constipation is causing fecal incontinence, dietary may recommend drinking plenty of fluids and eating fiber-rich foods. If diarrhea is contributing to the problem, high-fiber foods can also add bulk to stools and make them less watery [16]

The bowel is sensitive to the amount of fibre eaten, and also to contain foods. If a diet contains too much fibre the person may develop loose stools, if the diet is lacking in fibre, the person may become constipated. People who eat too much or too litttle fibre may develop FI. Certain foods, such as figs, prunes and plums, contain a natural laxative that can affect bowel habit. Some spices, such as chilli, can also affect the bowel. Excessive consumption of foods and drinks sweetened with sorbitol (an artificial sweetener) can cause loose stools [12].

A conscious effort to have a bowel movement at a specific time of day, for example, after eating. Establishing when you need to use the toilet can help you gain greater control [16].

Medications: If diarrhea is causing FI, medication may help. Health care providers sometimes recommend using bulk laxatives, such as Citrucel and Metamucil, to develop more solid stools that are easier to control. Antidiarrheal medications such as loperamide or diphenoxylate may be recommended to slow down the bowels and help control the problem [14]. If chronic constipation is causing FI, Laxatives may use [16].

Skin should be protected from Fecal enzymes by using either a barrier cream, such as Proshield Plus Skin Protective or Sudocrem", or a barier film such as Cavilon no sting barrier film [12].

Kegel exercises and biofeedback: Kegels or pelvic floor exercises can be problematic in frail older people who often have impaired cognition [12], but specially trained physiotherapists teach simple exercises that can increase anal muscle strength. People learn how to strengthen pelvic floor muscles, sense when stool is ready to be released and contract the muscles if having a bowel movement at a certain time is inconvenient. To perform Kegel exercises, contract the muscles that you would normally use to stop the flow of urine and stool. Hold the contraction for three seconds, then relax for three seconds. Repeat this pattern 10 times. As your muscles strengthen, hold the contraction longer, gradually working your way up to three sets of 10 contractions every day [16].

If the biofeedback session is aimed at strengthening your pelvic muscles, the practitioner will insert a slim sensor into your rectum. (In women, it is sometimes placed in the vagina, or an additional sensor may be used there.) Other electrodes will be placed on your abdomen to help record muscle contractions there. A computer screen provides feedback about the strength of your contractions and about whether you are using the correct muscles. If the biofeedback training is aimed at improving your ability to sense stool in the rectum, the practitioner will use anorectal manometry equipment to vary the pressure in your rectum. This is intended to increase the sensitivity of the rectum, which, in turn, helps some patients to recognize the presence of stool before the situation becomes despereat [17].

Surgery: Surgery may be an option for FI that fails to improve with other treatments or for FI caused by pelvic floor or anal sphincter muscle injuries [15].

Sphincteroplasty the most common FI surgery, reconnects the separated ends of a sphincter muscle torn by childbirth or another injury. Sphincteroplasty is performed at a hospital by a colorectal, gynecological or general surgeon [15].

Artificial anal sphincter involves placing an inflatable cuff around the anus and implanting a small pump beneath the skin that the person activates to inflate or deflate the cuff. This surgery is much less common and is performed at a hospital by a specially trained colorectal surgeon [18].

Nonabsorbable bulking agents can be injected into the wall of the anus to bulk up the tissue around the anus. The bulkier tissues make the opening of the anus narrower so the sphincters are able to close better. The procedure is performed in a health care provider's office; anesthesia is not needed. The person can return to normal physical activities 1 week after the procedure [18].

Bowel diversion: It is an operation that reroutes the normal movement of stool out of the body when part of the bowel is removed. The operation diverts the lower part of the small intestine or colon to an opening in the wall of the abdomen, the area between the chest and hips. An external pouch is attached to the opening to collect stool. The procedure is performed by a surgeon in a hospital and anesthesia is used [2-18].

Rectal irrigation: can be very benefical for some patients [12].

Colostomy: It is generally considered only after other treatments have been tried [16].

6. Fecal containment devices

Containment products, such as incontinence pads and pants, are widely used to collect feaces and provide a degree of protection, but should only be considered once all other treatment options have been explored [7].

Incontinance pads are not ideal when a person is FI with profuse diarrhoea or loose stools. In these cases, Fecal containment device may be appropriate, such as Dignicare (Bard) or Flexi-Seal (Convatec) [12].

Fecal containment device (FCD) prevents contact of perineal skin with fecal matter, reducing the risk for incontinence-associated dermatitis, pressure ulcer formation, fecal contamination of wounds and reduction in frequency of diaper, clothing, and linen changes [19].

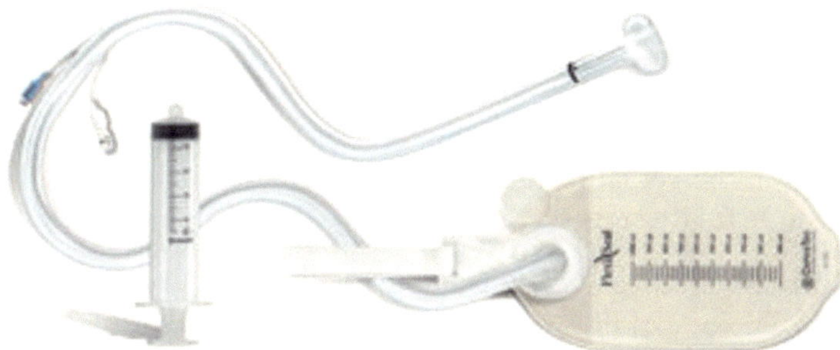

Figure 2. Fecal containment device [20].

FCD is an external drainage pouch that fits over the anus to collect stool. FCD and a bowel waste management system (BMS), which consists of an indwelling rectal catheter through which liquid or semi-liquid stool passes and is drained into an external drainage pouch. This patients should monitoring fluid and electrolyte status [20].

FCD, nurses responsibilities involved in the placement and maintenance of an FCD, including application (and removal) of the FCD based on the treating clinician's orders and manufacturer's instructions, the treating clinician's orders for the FCD, including pre-procedure analgesia. Any allergies; uses alternate materials during the procedure if allergies (e.g., latex) are noted [20].

7. Nursing care

1. In a reasonably private setting, directly question any patient at risk about the presence of FI. If the client reports altered bowel elimination patterns, problems with bowel control or "uncontrollable diarrhea," complete a focused nursing history including previous and present bowel elimination routines, dietary history, frequency and volume of uncontrolled stool loss, and aggravating and alleviating factors. Unless questioned directly, patients are unlikely to report the presence of FI [21]. The nursing history determines the patterns of stool elimination to characterize involuntary stool loss and the likely etiology of thein continence [22].

2. Complete a focused physical assessment including inspection of perineal skin, pelvic muscle strength assessment, digital examination of the rectum for presence of impaction and anal sphincter strength, and evaluation of functional status (mobility, dexterity, visual acuity).

   A focused physical examination helps determine the severity of fecal leakage and its likely etiology. A functional assessment provides information concerning the impact of functional status on stool elimination patterns and incontinence [23,24].

1. Complete an assessment of cognitive function. Dementia, acute confusion, and mental retardation are risk factors for FI [22,25].

2. Document patterns of stool elimination and incontinent episodes via a bowel record, including frequency of bowel movements, stool consistency, frequency and severity of incontinent episodes, precipitating factors, and dietary and fluid intake. This document is used to confirm the verbal history and to assist in determining the likely etiology of stool incontinence. It also serves as a baseline to evaluate treatment efficacy [22].

3. Identify the probable causes of FI. FI is frequently multifactorial; therefore identification of the probable etiology of FI is necessary to select a treatment plan likely to control or eliminate the condition [22,25,26].

4. Improve access to toileting:

   - Identify usual toileting patterns among persons in the acute care or long term care facility and plan opportunities for toileting accordingly.

   - Provide assistance with toileting for patients with limited access or impaired functional status (e.g., mobility, dexterity, access).

http://dx.doi.org/10.5772/57502

- Institute a prompted toileting program for persons with impaired cognitive status (e.g., retardation, dementia).
- Provide adequate privacy for toileting.
- Respond promptly to requests for assistance with toileting.
- Acute or transient FI frequently occurs in the acute care or long term care facility because of inadequate access to toileting facilities, insufficient assistance with toileting, or inadequate privacy when attempting to toilet [10,23,26,27].

5. For the patient with intermittent episodes of FI related to acute changes in stool consistency, begin a bowel reeducation program consisting of:

- Cleansing the bowel of impacted stool if indicated.
- Normalizing stool consistency by adequate intake of fluids (30ml/kg of body weight/ day) and dietary or supplemental fiber.
- Establishing a regular routine of fecal elimination based on established patterns of bowel elimination (patterns established before onset of incontinence).
- Bowel reeducation is designed to reestablish normal defecation patterns and to normalize stool consistency to reduce or eliminate the risk of recurring FI associated with changes in stool consistency [10].

6. Begin a prompted defecation program for the adult with dementia, mental retardation, or related learning disabilities. Prompted urine and fecal elimination programs have been shown to reduce or eliminate incontinence in the long term care facility and community settings [10,27].

7. Begin a scheduled stimulation defecation program, including the following steps, for persons with neurological conditions causing FI:

- Before beginning the program, cleanse the bowel of impacted fecal material.
- Implement strategies to normalize stool consistency, including adequate intake of fluid and fiber and avoidance of foods associated with diarrhea.
- Whenever feasible, determine a regular schedule for bowel elimination (typically every day or every other day) based on previous patterns of bowel elimination.
- Provide a stimulus before assisting the patient to a position on the toilet. Digital stimulation, stimulating suppository, "mini-enema," or pulsed evacuation enema may be used.
- The scheduled, stimulated defecation program relies on consistency of stool and a mechanical or chemical stimulus to produce a bolus contraction of the rectum with evacuation of fecal material [10,24,27].

8. Begin a pelvic floor reeducation or muscle exercise program for persons with sphincter incompetence or pseudodyssynergia of the pelvic muscles, or refer persons with fecal incontinence related to sphincter dysfunction to a nurse specialist or other therapist with clinical expertise in these techniques of care. Pelvic muscle reeducation, including biofeedback, pelvic muscle exercise, and/or pelvic muscle relaxation techniques, is a safe and effective treatment for selected persons with FI related to sphincter or pelvic floor muscle days function [23,26,27].

9. Begin a pelvic muscle biofeedback program among patients with urgency to defecate and FI related to recurrent diarrhea. Pelvic muscle reeducation, including biofeedback, can reduce uncontrolled loss of stool among persons who experience urgency and diarrhea as provacative factors for FI [28]. Reducing the incidence of diarrhea can help to reduce bowel incontinence [10,23].

10. Cleanse the perineal and perianal skin following each episode of FI. When incontinence is frequent, use an incontinence cleansing product specifically designed for this purpose. Frequent cleaning with soap and water, dry as possible may compromise perianal skin integrity and enhance the irritation produced by fecal leakage [1,29].

11. Apply mineral oil or a petroleum based ointment to the perianal skin when frequent episodes of FI occur. These products form a moisture and chemical barrier to the perianal skin that may prevent or reduce the severity of compromised skin integrity with severe FI [28].

12. Assist the patient to select and apply a containment device for occasional episodes of FI. A fecal containment device will prevent soiling of clothing and reduce odors in the patient with uncontrolled stool loss [28].

13. Teach the caregivers of the patient with frequent episodes of FI and limited mobility to regularly monitor the sacrum and perineal area for pressure ulcerations.Limited mobility, particularly when combined with FI, increases the risk of pressure ulceration. Routine cleansing, pressure reduction techniques, and management of fecal and urinary incontinence reduces this risk [23,24,21].

14. Consult the physician concerning the use of an anal continence plug for the patient with frequent stool loss. The anal continence plug is a device that can reduce or eliminate persistent liquid or solid stool incontinence in selected patients [18,28].

15. Apply a fecal pouch to the patient with frequent stool loss, particularly when FI produces altered perianal skin integrity. Fecal pouches contain stool loss, reduce odor, and protect the perianal skin from chemical irritation resulting from contact with stool [14,23].

16. Consult the physician concerning the use of a rectal tube for the patient with severe FI. A large-sized French indwelling catheter has been used for fecal containment when incontinence is severe and perianal skin integrity significantly compromised [26].

http://dx.doi.org/10.5772/57502

8. Evidence — Based practices in fecal incontinence

Evidence Based Practice (EBP) is the use of systematic decision-making processes or provision of services which have been shown, through available scientific evidence, to consistently improve measurable patient outcomes. Instead of tradition, gut reaction or single observations as the basis for making decisions, EBP relies on data collected through experimental research and accounts for individual patient characteristics and clinician expertise.

Evidence Based Treatments (EBTs) are interventions which have scientific findings to demonstrate their effectiveness or efficacy in improving patient outcomes. Treatments are often placed along a continuum of support based on the rigorousness and amount of supporting research ranging from treatments which have strong support to those which are untested to those which have produced negative outcomes. Data sources used to make these evidence determinations include randomized experiments, which compare treatment with a control or placebo group or compare the treatment with another already established treatment; and single case design experiments which compare an individual subject's baseline with their response to treatment [30].

There are four or five generally accepted evidence levels along the continuum of research support on which experts attempt to categorize practices, based on the body of evidence and outcomes indicated supporting each treatment method.

A. Evidence of Type I or consistent findings from multiple studies of Type II, III, or IV
B. Evidence of Type II, III, or IV and generally consistent findings
C. Evidence of Type II, III, or IV but inconsistent findings
D. Little or no systematic empirical evidence

Table 3. Grades of Recommendations [31]

I. Meta-analysis of multiple well-designed, controlled studies, randomized trials with low false- positive and low false-negative errors (high power).
II. At least one well-designed experimental study; randomized trials with high false-positive or high false-negative errors or both (low power).
III. Well-designed, quasi-experimental studies, such as nonrandomized, controlled, single-group, preoperative-postoperative comparison, cohort, time, or matched case-control series.
IV. Well-designed, nonexperimental studies, such as cornparative and correlational descriptive and case studies.
V. Case reports and clinical examples.

Table 4. Levels of Evidence [31]

	Level of Evidence	Grade of Recommendation
Assessment		
1. Evaluation of FI should include consideration of severity and impact.	**Class II**	**B**
Diagnosis		
1. A problem-specific history and physical examination should be performed.	**Class V**	**D**
2. Endoanal ultrasound is usually the procedure of choice to diagnose sphincter defects in patients with suspected sphincter injury. Anorectal physiology studies mav be helpful in guiding management.	**Class II**	**B**
Nonoperative Treatment		
1. A trial of increased fiber intake is recommended in milder forms of FI to improve symptoms.	**Class III**	**B**
2. Antidiarrheal agents, such as adsorbents or opium derivatives, mav reduce FI symptoms.	**Class III**	**C**
3. Enemas, laxatives, and suppositories mav help to promote more complete bowel emptying in appropriate patients and minimize further postdefecation leakage	**Class V**	**D**
4. Biofeedback is recommended as an initial treatment for motivated patients with incontinence with some voluntary sphincter contraction.	**Class III**	**B**
5. An anal plug is effective in controlling FI in a smail minority of patients who can tolerate its use.	**Class V**	**D**
Surgical Options		
1.Sphincter repair is appropriately offered to highly symptomatic patients with a defined defect of the external anal sphincter.	**Class II**	**A**
2. Overlapping or direct sphincter repair yield similar results, as long as adequate mobilization of both ends of the sphincters are performed.	**Class II**	**A**
3. Repeat anal sphincter repair could be considered in patients who have recurrent symptoms and residual anterior sphincter defect after a previous sphincter repair.	**Class III**	**B**
4. Repair of the internal anal sphincter alone has a poor functional outcome and is not generally recommended.	**Class III**	**B**
5. When passiye FI caused by internal sphincter dysfunction is the predominant symptom, injectable therapy seems to be effective and safe, although its long-term efficacy has yet to be defined.	**Class II**	**B**
6.Sacral nerve stimulation (SNS) is a promising modality for FI.	**Class III**	**B**
7. Postanal repair or total pelvic floor repair has a limited role in the treatment of neuropathic FI.	**Class III**	**B**
8. Dynamic graciloplasty mav have a role in the treatment of severe FI when there is irreparable sphincter disruption.	**Class III**	**B**
9. The artificial bowel sphincter has a role in the treatment of severe FI, especially in patients with significant sphincter disruption.	**Class III**	**B**
10. The SECCA (safety and effectiveness of temperature-controlled radiofrequency energy delivery to the anal canal) procedure mav be useful for selected patients with moderate FI.	**Class IV**	**C**
11. A stoma (colostomy or ileostomy) is appropriate for patients with limiting FI in which available treatments have failed, are inappropriate because of comorbidities, or when preferred by the patient.	**Class III**	**B**

Table 5. Evidence- Based Practices İn Fecal İncontinence [31]

8.1. Assessment

Severity instruments assess type, frequency, and amount of incontinence. Impact questionnaires address quality of life and attempt to evaluate the effect of incontinence on emotional, occupational, physical, and social function. Both should evaluate these relatively subjective factors with reliability and validity [31].

8.2. Diagnosis

A detailed medical history mav help to elicit contributing or exacerbating factors, such as gastrointestinal or neurologic disorders. An obstetric account or history of previous anorectal surgery or perineal trauma can direct/prompt a more focused examination.

Inspection of the perianal skin may reveal excoriation, surgical scars, or fistulas, and the anus mav be noted to gape upon spreading the buttocks. Mucosal or full-thickness prolapse may be elicited with a Valsalva maneuver. Digital examination mav provide a rough estimate of resting and squeeze pressures and is helpful to evaluate for a rectal mass or the presence of impacted stool, which would suggest overflow as a possible mechanism for incontinence. Anoscopy and flexible sigmoidoscopy mav help to identify hemorrhoids, inflammatory bowel disease, or neoplasms [31].

8.3. Nonoperative treatment

Nonoperative therapy is usually the first maneuver to improve the symptoms of FI. Most patients with mild FI should usually receive an initial trial of nonoperative management.

Gradual increase of fiber intake during a period of several days can reduce symptoms, such as abdominal bloating and discomfort that mav be associated with increased fiber intake. Fiber supplements in the form of powder, granule, or pill of ten facilitate this goal. Dairy products are problematic in patients with lactose intolerance.

Antidiarrheal agents, adsorbents, such as kaopectate (Pharmacia & Upjohn, Peapack, NJ), act by absorbing excess fluid in the stool. Commonly used opium derivatives are loperamide (Imodium, McNeil Consumer Healthcare, Fort Washington, PA), diphenoxylate hydrochloride plus atropine sulphate (Lomotil, Searle, Chicago, IL), codeine, and tincture of opium. Evaluation and management of abnormal colonic transit also can be helpful.

Biofeedback mav be considered a first-line option for many patients with FI who have not responded to simple dietary modification or medication.

Supportive counseling and practical advice regarding diet and skin care can improve the success of biofeedback. Biofeedback mav be considered before attempting sphincter repair or for those who have persistent or recurrent symptoms after sphincter repair. it mav have a role in the early postpartum period in females with symptomatic sphincter weakness. Biofeedback and a pelvic floor exercise program can produce improvement that lasts more than two years. Biofeedback home training is an alternative to ambulatory training programs, especially in the elderly [31].

8.4. Surgical options

The SECCA (safety and effectiveness of temperature-controlled radiofrequency energy delivery to the anal canal) procedure consists of the delivery of temperature-controlled radiofrequency energy to the anal sphincters. It is believed that the heat generated causes collagen contraction, healing, and remodeling, leading to shorter and tighter muscle fibers [31].

Author details

Arzu Ilce*

Address all correspondence to: arzuilce@hotmail.com

Abant Izzet Baysal University, Bolu Health School, Department of Nursing Turkish, Bolu, Turkey

References

[1] Jarrett ME, Mowatt G, Glazener CM, et al. Systematic review of sacral nerve stimulation for fecal incontinence and constipation. Br J Surg 2004; 91:1559.

[2] Rao SS, American College of Gastroenterology Practice Parameters Committee. Diagnosis and management of fecal incontinence. American College of Gastroenterology Practice Parameters Committee. Am J Gastroenterology 2004; 99:1585.

[3] Barnett JL, Hasler WL, Camilleri M. American Gastroenterological Association medical position statement on anorectal testing techniques. American Gastroenterological Association. Gastroenterology 2009; 116:732.

[4] Caple C, Cabrera G, Strayer DA, Incontinence, Fecal, in Women, Editor Diane Pravikoff, Cinahl Information Systems, May 6, 2011

[5] Harvie HS, Arya LA, Saks EK, et al. Utility preference score measurement in women with fecal incontinence. Am J Obstet Gynecol 2011;204:721-726.

[6] Markland AD, Richter HE, Burgio KL, et al. Fecal incontinence in obese women with urinary incontinence: prevalence and role of dietary fiber intake. Am J Obstet Gynecol 2009;200:5661-5666.

[7] Woodward S, Management options for Fecal incontinence. Nursing & Residential Care 2012; 14: 5.

[8] Bliss DZ and Norton C, Conservative Management of Fecal Incontinence. AJN 2010; 110: 9.

[9] Madoff RD, Williams JG, Caushaj PF. Fecal incontinence. N Engl J Med 1999;326:1002-07.

[10] Wong WD, Congliosi SM, Spencer MP, et al. The safety and efficacy of the artificial bowel sphincter for fecal incontinence: results from a multicenter cohort study. Dis Colon Rectum 2002;45:1139–53.

[11] Whitehead WE, Borrud L, Goode PS, et al. Fecal incontinence in U.S. adults: epidemiology and risk factors. Gastroenterology.2009;137(2):512-17.

[12] Nazarko L, Fecal incontinence: diagnosis, treatmentandmanagement. Nursing & Residential Care. 2011;13(6):270-5

[13] Cabot Health, Bristol Stool Chart http://www.cabothealth.com.au/articles/bristol-stool-chart-2/ (accessed 30 november 2013)

[14] Keating JP, Stewart PJ, Eyers AA, et al. Are special investigations of value in the management of patients with fecal incontinence? Dis Colon Rectum 2012 ; 40:896.

[15] Slavin JL. Position of the American Dietetic Association: health implications of dietary fiber. Journal of the American Dietetic Association.2008;108(31):1716–1731.

[16] Mayo Clinic, Fecal İncontinence, http://www.mayoclinic.com/health/fecal-incontinence/DS00477 (accessed 30 november 2013)

[17] Harvard Health PublicationS, Better Bladder and Bowel Control, 38- 41, www.health,harvard.edu (accessed 30 november 2013)

[18] Ko CY, Tong J, Lehman RE, et al. Biofeedback is effective therapy for fecal incontinence and constipation. Arch Surg 2010; 132:829.

[19] Schub E, Fecal Containment Devices: Providing Patient Care. Cinahl Information Systems 2012.

[20] Fecal containment device http://www.convatec.com/continence-critical-care/flexi-seal-family-of-products/flexi-seal-fms.aspx (accessed 30 november 2013)

[21] Duel BP, Gonzalez R. The button cecostomy for management of fecal incontinence. Pediatr Surg Int 1999;15(8):559-61.

[22] Norton C, Chelvanayagam S, Wilson-Barnett J, et al. Randomized controlled trial of biofeedback for fecal incontinence. Gastroenterology 2003;125:1320-29.

[23] Gray M, Burns SM. Continence management. Crit Care Nurs Clinics N Am 1996;8(1): 29-38.

[24] Fynes M, O'Herlihy C. The influence of mode of delivery on anal sphincter injury and fecal continence. The Obstetrician Gynaecologist 2001;3:120–25.

[25] Jensen LL, Lowry AC. Biofeedback improves functional outcome after sphincteroplasty. Dis Colon Rectum 1997;40(2):197-200

[26] Wald A. Biofeedback for neurogenic fecal incontinence: Rectal sensation is a determinant of outcome. J Pediatr Gastoenterol Nutr 2005;2:302-06.

[27] Shafik A. Perianal injection of autologous fat for treatment of sphincteric incontinence. Dis Colon Rectum 1995;38:583-87.

[28] Chiang L, Ouslander J, Schnelle J, et al. Dually incontinent nursing home residents: Clinical characteristics and treatment differences. J Am Geriatr Soc 2000;48(6):673–76.

[29] Alstad B, Sahlin Y, Myrvold HE. Anal plug in fecal incontinence. Tidsskrift for Den Norske Laegeforening 1999;119(3):365-66.

[30] Evidence Based Practice Institute http://depts.washington.edu/ebpi/ (accessed 30 november 2013)

[31] National Guideline Clearinghause, http://www.guideline.gov/search/search.aspx?term=fecal+incontinence (accessed 24 september 2013)

Chapter 3

Anal Incontinence as a Complication of Vaginal Delivery and Anorectal Surgery

Małgorzata Kołodziejczak and
Iwona Sudoł-Szopińska

Additional information is available at the end of the chapter

http://dx.doi.org/10.5772/57358

1. Introduction

Incontinence is a complex term and encompasses a broad spectrum of disorders with various intensities. They range from gas incontinence, through incontinence of liquid stools (soiling), to incontinence of solid stools.

The factors determining the function of faecal continence comprise: structural elements such as the anal sphincter muscles and pelvic floor muscles, including the Parks angle (between the long axis of the rectum and that of the anal canal), as well as functional elements such as central nervous system, anorectal sensation, volume and compliance of the rectum, stool consistency, high-pressure zone and abdominal pressure.

Faecal incontinence affects 2-7% of the adult population. The range of the problem is not exactly known due to its embarrassing nature and reluctance to report stool and/or gas incontinence to physicians [1, 2, 3]. The majority of patients are women. It has been reported that 1 on 10 women suffers from various types of incontinence [4], the most common cause being obstetric trauma (60%). The second most common cause is iatrogenic injury to the anal sphincter muscles sustained during anorectal surgeries (approximately 16%) [5, 6]. More and more often, incontinence is caused by injuries that occur after inserting foreign bodies to the rectum and after traffic injuries. The number of patients with inflammatory bowel diseases is rising as well. Neurogenic incontinence is also a contributor [7]. This chapter discusses two groups of causes: obstetric and those occurring after anorectal surgery.

2. Obstetric anal sphincter defects

Obstetric trauma is the most common cause of faecal incontinence in women. Symptoms of incontinence that persist for more than 6 months after the delivery are reported by ¼ of women. The number is even higher in primiparas [8].

Risk factors for post-partum faecal incontinence may generally be divided into those dependent on the mother and the course of the labour itself, and those related to the child. The most significant risk factors related to the mother and the course of labour are: occurrence of a third- or fourth-degree perineal tear, instrumental delivery, primiparity, age of the mother, number of previous deliveries, duration of the second stage of labour, application of epidural anaesthesia, oxytocin in the second stage of labour and breech delivery [9, 10]. The most commonly identified child-related risk factors include an excessively heavy infant and large head circumference. A strong correlation between fetal macrosomia and anal sphincter defects of the mother as well as injuries during labour was confirmed by Gumundson et al. [11]. Amongst all these aforementioned risk factors, the most significant is the occurrence of either a third- or fourth-degree perineal tear.

There are several classifications of obstetric anal sphincter injuries. One of them distinguishes evident and occult anal sphincter defects on clinical examination. Evident obstetric injuries of the anal sphincters are diagnosed by an obstetrician during suturing the perineum. They encompass third- and fourth-degree perineal tears, i.e. those which involve the anal sphincters (third-degree defects) or in addition, encompass the rectal mucus membrane (four-degree defects).

An additional division of third-degree perineal tears [12] includes the size of sphincteric defects i.e.:

- First degree. The rupture encompasses less than 50% of the thickness of the external anal sphincter.
- Second degree. The rupture encompasses more than 50% of the thickness of the external anal sphincter.
- Third degree. The rupture encompasses the external and internal anal sphincters.

Occult obstetric defects constitute cases that are not diagnosed directly after the delivery when the perineum is sutured. These defects are not usually accompanied by changes in the perineal region, which is the main reason for the failure to diagnose them by an obstetrician. In our own research, the percentage of detected defects after natural delivery reached 3.9% [3].The symptomatic presentation of sphincteric insufficiency connected with occult defects is usually delayed, sometimes up to a dozen years after the delivery. This is probably because such injuries are less extensive than in evident cases.

Another classification of obstetric defects is their division into structural (or mechanical) injuries and neurogenic incontinence.

3. Obstetric mechanical (structural) defects

Mechanical injuries of the anal sphincters encompass the complete or incomplete disruption of the external or internal anal sphincters (Figure 1 a, b).

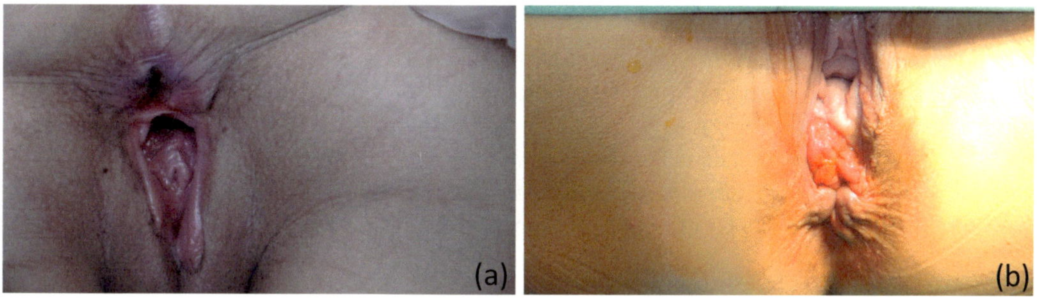

Figure 1. a) An obstetric tear of anal sphincters; b) an obstetric tear of anal sphincters with a rupture of the rectovaginal septum

The anatomy of the anal sphincters in women predisposes them to such injuries. In men the entire length of the anal anterior wall in made up of two muscle layers corresponding to internal and external sphincters. In contrast, in the majority of women, the external sphincter is not present in the superior aspect of the anal canal on the anterior wall. Traumatic vaginal deliveries occur particularly frequently in women in whom the distance between the fourchette and the anal canal is short.

Mechanical injuries of the sphincters are not always accompanied by incontinence. In younger women, obstetric injuries may be compensated by the function of the remaining, retained mass of the sphincters, mainly by the puborectalis muscle. By creating the, so-called, Parks angle between the anus and rectum, this is a crucial muscle responsible for continence [13]. Symptoms of sphincteric insufficiency may eventually develop in the menopausal period when the pelvic floor muscles weaken, pudendal nerve neuropathy occurs.

4. Obstetric neurogenic incontinence

Neurogenic injuries are primarily occur during delivery of a large fetus. A prolonged second stage of labour lasting more than 60 minutes results in prolonged compression of the pudendal nerves by the fetal head (the nerve is pressed against the ischial spine). The nerve may also become irreversibly damaged when it is exposed to pressures of more than 80 mmHg for more than 8 hours [14]. Prolonged bearing down may stretch the pelvic floor structures, including the pudendal nerves. This disruption may involve branches of the spinal roots in the sacral spine S3-4 which run on the internal aspect of the pelvic floor and innervate, among others, the puborectalis muscle.

The second stage of labour, lasting from full cervical dilation to the delivery, is considered the most traumatic for the pelvic floor muscles, including the sphincters [14]. In this period, the muscles and tissues of the pelvic floor are subject to the greatest pressure, perineal descent is observed and directly after the delivery, transitory changes in the muscle tone may occur [15]. As many as 80% of women develop transient denervation of the pelvic floor [16,17]. Muscle fibres become mechanically damaged when they are stretched by more than 50% and the perineal nerve fibres undergo damage as a result of their stretching by 6-22% [18].

In prolonged labour, the pudendal nerve, which is compressed by the fetal head against the ischial spine, is the most susceptible to injuries. Snooks et al. [19] found evidence of prolonged latency of the pudendal nerve in as many as 48% of women within 48-72 hours following delivery. This was interpreted as a direct proof of injury. Damage to the pudendal nerve may cause not only faecal incontinence, but also urinary incontinence and sexual dysfunction. Obstetric injuries may also be mixed with both structural defects features of pudendal nerve neuropathy.

5. Anal sphincter defects following anorectal surgeries

Faecal incontinence may appear even after the simplest anal surgery. It may occur after haemorrhoidectomy as well as surgeries for anal fissures or fistulae.

5.1. Incontinence after haemorrhoidectomy

Classical haemorrhoidectomy may result in the inability to discriminate between the contents of the rectum with resulting incontinence. More rarely sphincteric defects can occur. Inability to discriminate between the nature of the rectal contents (anal sensation failure) results from too extensive excision of the mucus membrane that is rich in sensory receptors.

The receptors that differentiate between solid and liquid stools as well as gases are localised in the transitional zone which constitutes an area of approximately 1.5 cm in length situated over the dental line.

Pudendal nerve damage can also result in faecal urgency. This can occur after too extensive excision of haemorrhoids in the commonly employed Milligan-Morgan procedure. It may also occur following Longo's stapled haemorrhoidectomy if the stapler is placed too low, inadvertently resecting the entire transitional zone.

Haemorrhoidectomy may also result in mechanical injury of the sphincters, particularly the internal sphincter. "Post PPH syndrome" has been reported when the staplers are placed slightly low, possibly causing the internal sphincter muscle to become inflamed.

5.2. Incontinence after anal fissure surgery

One of the main reasons for the appearance of anal fissure is increased tension with subsequent hypertrophy of the internal anal sphincter. Anorectal manometry has identified a considerably higher mean maximum resting pressure in the anal canal (reflecting mainly internal sphincter function) in patients with anal fissures as compared with controls [20].

Anal fissure surgery always requires cutting the sphincter responsible for the continence of gases and liquid stools. It has been estimated that faecal incontinence occurs after anal fissure surgery in 3-38% patients [21]. The surgical treatment of anal fissures includes the following methods: open and closed lateral sphincterotomy, open posterior sphincterotomy without excision of the fissure and open posterior sphincterotomy with excision of the fissure. Open lateral sphincterotomy is the gold standard for the management of chronic anal fissures [22]. The proportion developing postoperative incontinence when using this technique ranges from 0-16% [23, 24]. The surgical treatment of chronic or recurring fissures may involve techniques based on mucosal advancement flap anoplasty, anal advancement flap or anodermal flap [25, 26].

The most recent modification of lateral sphincterotomy is segmental internal sphincterotomy [27]. It appears that this type of surgery does not carry the risk of incontinence [27]. Another surgical treatment involves anal dilation with the use of either a Parks' anal retractor that is spread to 4.8 cm, or a rectosigmoid balloon 40 mm in diameter and 60 mm in length [28]. The effectiveness of this method is comparable to classical lateral sphincterotomy (83.3% and 92% respectively). Following 24 months of observation, no complications in the form of incontinence were observed in a group treated by means of the dilator [29].

Open posterior sphincterotomy, apart from the consequences resulting from cutting the internal sphincter, may also cause a "keyhole deformity" of the anal canal, resulting in anal leakage and soiling of the underwear.

Patients identified with increased pressure in the anal canal have been treated with botulinum toxin administered intersphincterically. Worsening of continence was not observed over a 24 month observation period, and only 8% of patients suffered a relapse [26].

5.3. Incontinence after anal fistula surgeries

Anal fistula surgery nearly always results in the controlled severing of anal sphincter muscles. The risk of incontinence increases with so-called height of the fistula (the length of the external anal sphincter involved by the fistula), its localisation in relation to the wall of the anal canal (anterior fistulae in women), recurring fistulae and coexistence of a neurogenic component in addition to the morphological defect.

The most common cause of incontinence after anal fistula surgery is from extensive damage of the sphincter muscles sustained during the course of the procedure (Figure 2).

Reasons for sphincteric damage include:

- overly aggressive surgical techniques in patients whose sphincteric function was impaired before surgery;
- incorrect intraoperative assessment of the type of fistula and inappropriate surgical method;

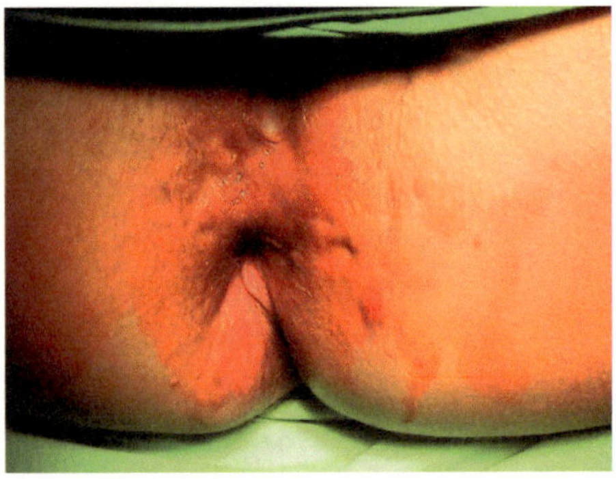

Figure 2. Iatrogenic anal sphincter injury following fistulectomy

- setons kept in the wound for too long, resulting in fibrosis of the sphincter muscles and worsening gas and stool continence;
- anal canal deformation (keyhole deformity), which often appears following the Hippocratic method of treatment and may lead to faecal soiling;- bilateral damage to the inferior anal nerves that innervate the external anal sphincter in the surgery of horseshoe abscesses or fistulae (a rare complication).

Patients with fistulae and abscesses accompanying non-specific inflammatory bowel disease can be particularly difficult cases.

The proportion developing postoperative incontinence depends on the surgical technique. Following fistulotomy, worsening of continence is observed in as many as 45% of patients [30, 31] and following fistulotomy with sphincter reconstruction - from 4 to 32% of cases [32, 33, 34]. Incontinence is hardly ever observed after direct closure of the internal fistula opening.

Treatment of the internal orifice of the fistula by endorectal advancement flap results in postoperative incontinence in 13.2% of cases [35]. Methods involving anal fistula plugs or fibrin glue introduced to the fistula canal do not cause gas and stool incontinence, but a high percentage of relapse is observed [36]. Cutting seton fistulotomy is not currently recommended since the rate of continence disorders after this procedure reaches 90% [37, 38].

The risk of incontinence resulting from surgical treatment of fistulae can be minimised by assessing sphincteric sufficiency by means of anorectal manometry. It is also important to identify the position of the fistula in relation to the sphincters by means of supplementary examinations such as anorectal endosonography or MRI.

6. Diagnosis and treatment of obstetric and postoperative anal sphincter defects

The general procedures performed in obstetric and postoperative incontinence are similar. All patients after anorectal surgeries and all women after third- or fourth-degree perineal tear should undergo a rectal examination and endosonographic scan. Additionally, in the case of faecal incontinence symptoms, functional tests should also be performed. Repairing obstetric sphincter defects should be treated in the same way as repair surgeries of any other types of sphincteric damage since improper suturing of the muscles with ongoing functional failure by the sutured muscles may result in permanent disablement. The costs of treatment of remote complications are higher than the costs of preventive diagnostic examinations.

6.1. Diagnosis of obstetric and postoperative anal sphincter defects

Diagnosis of incontinence requires doctor-patient interview, anorectal examination, functional tests and imaging examinations particularly endosonography and magnetic resonance imaging.

Interview

The interview and physical rectal examinations are the basic methods for diagnosing and formulating treatment of incontinence.

Patients should be asked about the presence of underwear soiling, uncontrollable passage of gasses or stools as well as about the nature of such symptoms (temporary or permanent) and the frequency with which they occur. Female patients should be asked about their deliveries (instrumental delivery, episiotomy, fetal size, duration of labour etc.). It is important to find out whether incontinence is related to other factors (e.g. physical effort or stress), if there has been previous anorectal surgery or whether there are coexistant diseases that might affect continence such as neurological conditions, lumbosacral discopathies or inflammatory bowel diseases. An objective assessment of the symptoms can be provided through various scoring systems for the evaluation of anal sphincteric insufficiency which also include subjective elements (e.g. Wexner score) [39]. Quality of Life tests are also available (e.g. Fecal Incontinence Quality of Life) [40].

6.1.1. Anorectal examination

Visual examination of the anal region enables identification of post-surgical scarring, anal deformities and episiotomy scars.

During digital anorectal examination, one should assess passive and active tone of the sphincters and content of the anus. It is also possible to determine the site of the external sphincter defect by asking the patient to contract the sphincters. Nevertheless, some studies report that the percentage of sphincteric defects detectable by means of a clinical examination does not exceed 50% [41].

6.1.2. Functional test

From the point of view of possible surgical treatment, the most useful supplementary examination is anorectal manometry. This allows determination of anorectal function by measuring resting and squeeze pressure in the anal canal as well as other significant parameters such as: cough reflex, manometric changes during attempted defecation, rectoanal inhibitory reflex, rectal sensation, high pressure zone length, functional sphincter length, and basic rectosphincteric reflexes for instance, rectoanal inhibitory reflex (RAIR).

Anorectal manometry can be particularly useful when surgeries, e.g. of anal fistulae [42], are planned and before sphincter repair procedures. The effectiveness of sphincteric repair surgeries is not always satisfactory and functional documentation of the sphincters from before the procedure is crucial not only for medical but also legal reasons.

Another useful functional test is electromyography. This determines the myoelectrical activity of the sphincters when resting, during contraction and during faecal urgency. The examination can be performed invasively with the use of thin concentric needle electrodes placed in the lateral fragments of the sphincter around and parallel to the anal canal. It can also be performed in a less invasive manner with the use of superficial cutaneous electromyography and for instance a 16-channel probe [43]. Other functional examinations are of less importance.

Pelvic floor descent may be visualised by means of conventional defecography as well as in dynamic MRI. It provides a comprehensive evaluation of the lateral and anterior aspects of the pelvic floor while resting and during urgency and involves the introduction of water, gel or solution with contrast agent (depending on the experience of the centre) into the lumen of the bladder, vagina or rectum (dynamic MR colpocystorectography). This examination enables assessment of pelvic floor motility.

6.1.3. Imaging examinations

The imaging examination of choice in patients with incontinence symptoms is anal endosonography (AES). The primary aim of AES is to differentiate between the causes of incontinence: whether there is evidence of morphological injury of the sphincters as might be expected in a tear or whether the features are more consistent with a neurogenic cause. In the case of neurogenic incontinence, the sphincters may appear normal or atrophic, and during attempted sphincter contraction as part of a dynamic AES there is no evidence of contraction of the external sphincter and puborectalis muscle. This examination should be performed prior to planned anal and rectal surgeries in all patients who manifest symptoms of incontinence (in order to minimise further impairment of sphincteric function) as well as in patients who have already undergone anorectal surgeries but have postoperative incontinence, in order to explain its cause (Figure 3 a, b).

In the case of women who sustain labour-induced third- or fourth-degree injury to the perineum, AES is important to perform because of the asymptomatic character of numerous injuries which may be compensated by the undamaged retained portion of the sphincters (Figure 4 a, b).

If defects are detected, one should determine:

- which muscle has been damaged (internal, external anal sphincter or puborectalis muscle);
- the range of damage (circumference and length in relation to anal canal levels);
- the presentation of the retained sphincters (muscle stumps).

http://dx.doi.org/10.5772/57358

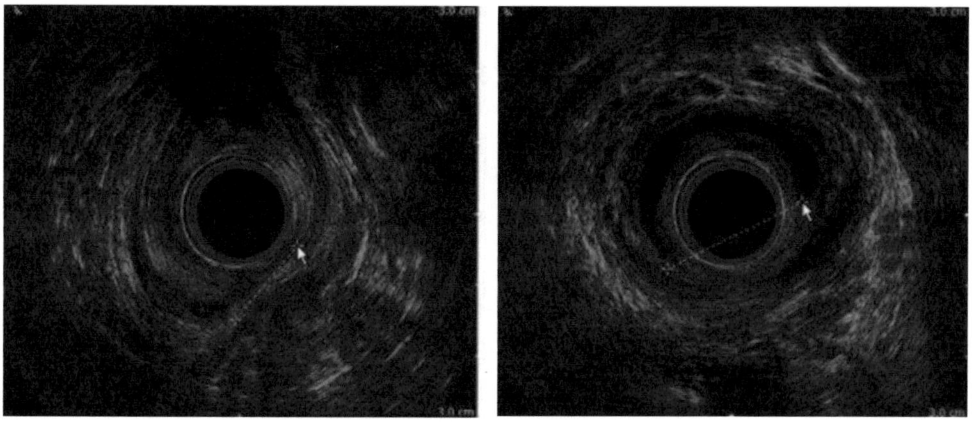

Figure 3. External and internal anal sphincter tears following fistulectomy due to posterior transsphincteric fistula surgery, affecting: a) in a distal part of the anal canal 30% of the posterior-right circumference of the external anal sphincter; b) in mid anal level 50% of the posterior aspect of the internal anal sphincters. Muscle stumps are normal

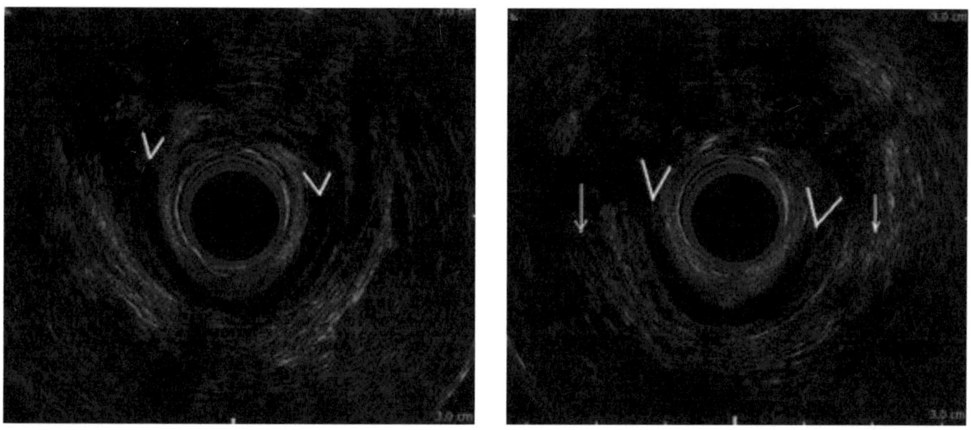

Figure 4. Obstetric structural defect of anal sphincters in AES: a) high anal canal level with an anterior tear of the 30% of the internal anal sphincter circumference (dashes); b) mid anal canal level with an anterior tear of the 50% of the internal and external anal sphincters circumference (arrows). Retained muscles are normal

Endosonographic examination is also performed to assist in the diagnosis of rectovaginal fistulae which frequently accompany obstetric sphincter defects (Figure 5).

Magnetic resonance imaging with the use of a torso/pelvic coil or endoanal coil is rarely used in the postoperative diagnosis of faecal incontinence because endosonography, which is cheaper and simpler, allows for good visualisation of the sphincters. However, the selection of diagnostic methods mainly depends on their accessibility, experience of the centre/examiner and costs of the examination (Figure 6).

Computed tomography, on the other hand, is not helpful in diagnosing anal sphincter defects because it does not allow for the discrimination between individual anal sphincters.

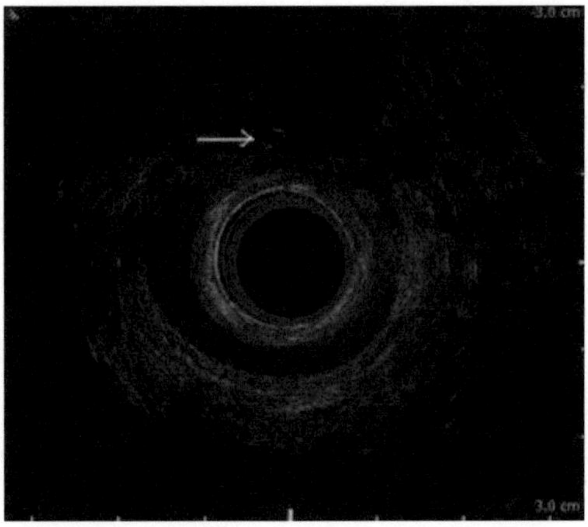

Figure 5. Obstetric ano-vaginal fistula in AES (arrow)

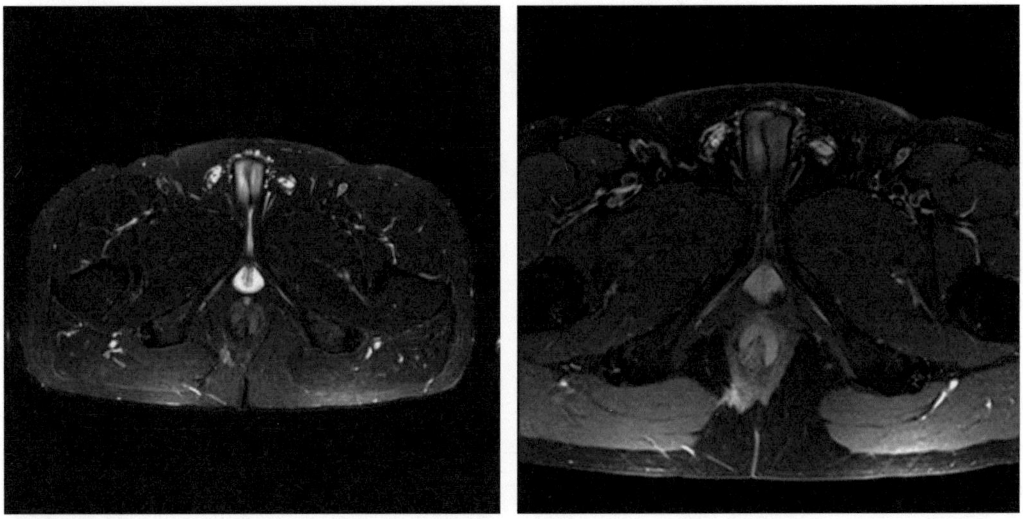

Figure 6. Posterior defect of the internal anal sphincter in: a) T2 TIRM and b) T1F2CE axial images following surgery for intersphincteric fistula

7. Treatment of obstetric and postoperative incontinence

The treatment of incontinence should be comprehensive and should take place in coloproctological referral centres.

7.1. Conservative treatment

In the majority of cases, conservative treatment is offered initially and encompasses a stool thickening diet, antidiarrheal medications, exercising sphincter muscles and pelvic floor muscles as well as electrostimulation of the sphincters with biofeedback. Psychological supervision is also essential in numerous patients.

The biofeedback method uses biological feedback i.e. enables patients to monitor the progress of their therapy by means of special devices which allow for the visual (change of colour) or auditory (sound) registration of the therapy progress (e.g. increasing contraction strength of the sphincters while exercising).

Electrostimulation of sphincters is performed with devices using endoanal electrodes. The effectiveness of such procedures is assessed in various ways. This, among others, results from the lack of uniform qualification criteria for such therapies.

7.2. Surgical treatment

The best functional effects are brought about by immediate suturing of the muscles directly after the trauma. This particularly refers to obstetric damage to the anal sphincters. If immediate repair is not possible (due to inexperienced team or occult damage) the therapeutic decision should be postponed until the tissues have healed [44].

Scheduled reconstruction of anal sphincters is burdened with a high risk of failure even in specialised referral centres. Prior to such procedures, it is crucial to conduct imaging and functional examinations of the anal sphincters in order to qualify the patient for the procedure. If the defect involves more than 30% of the anal circumference, the operator is forced to consider protective stoma. If, however, the sphincteric defect exceeds 50%, the repair surgery is practically certain to fail. When the damage to the external sphincter is partial (not involving the entire thickness), the muscles may be sutured by interrupted sutures (end-to-end repair) without mobilising the ends. If, however, the muscle is completely severed, the stumps should be mobilised and sutured by the overlapping technique. This method brings about the best outcomes.

Surgical treatment should be complemented with conservative therapy i.e. exercises strengthening the muscles and anorectal sensation (biofeedback) as well as electrical stimulation of the anal sphincters.

8. Conclusion

Incontinence is a condition of a multifactorial etiology. It is difficult to treat and requires specialised diagnosis. What is more, patients with faecal incontinence should remain under the supervision of a multidisciplinary team of physicians including specialists in fields such as surgical coloproctology, radiologists as well as psychologists. Diagnosis and treatment should take place in the centres specialising in coloproctology. Finally, rehabilitation of patients following sphincteric surgeries is essential and may considerably improve the ultimate outcome of the procedure.

Author details

Małgorzata Kołodziejczak[1*] and Iwona Sudoł-Szopińska[2,3]

*Address all correspondence to: drkolodziejczak@o2.pl

1 Department of Proctology, Hospital at Solec, Warsaw, Poland

2 Department of Radiology, Institute of Rheumatology, Warsaw, Poland

3 Department of Diagnostic Imaging, Warsaw Medical University, Warsaw, Poland

References

[1] Nelson RL. Epidemiology of fecal incontinence. Gastroenterology 2004;126(1): 3-7.

[2] Madoff RD. Fecal incontinence in adults. Lancet 2004;364: 621-32.

[3] Kołodziejczak M, Sudoł-Szopińska I, Stefański R, Panorska AK, Gardyszewska A, Krasnodębski I. Anal endosonographic findings in women after vaginal delivery. European Journal of Radiology 2011;78(1): 157-9.

[4] Bharucha AE, Zinsmeister AR, Locke GR, Seide BM, McKeon K, Schlec CD, Melton J. Prevalence and burden of fecal incontinence: a population-based study in women. Gastroenterology 2005;129: 42-9.

[5] Barthet M, Bellon P, Abou E, Portier F, Berdah S, Lesavre N, Orsoni P, Bouvier M, Grimaud JC. The International Journal of Colorectal Disease 2002;17(2): 123.

[6] Morris C, Osterweil P, Hong LI, Rosenberg D, Greenlick MN. Incidence of fecal incontinence after childbirth. Obstetrics & Gynecology 2007;109(1): 281-8.

[7] Satish S.C Rao Pathophysiology of adult fecal incontinence 2004;126: 14–22.

[8] Fitzpatrick M, O'Herlihy C. The effects of labour and delivery on the pelvic floor Best Practice and Research Clinical Obstetrics & Gynecology 2001;15: 63-79.

[9] Leuw JW, Struijk PC, Vierhout ME, Wallenburg HCS. Risk factors for third degree perineal ruptures during delivery. British Journal of Obstetrics and Gynaecology 2001;108: 383-7.

[10] De Parades V, Etienney I, Thabut D, Beaulieu S, Tawk M, Assemekang B, Marie V, Toubia ML, Wehbe A, Mosnier H, Gadonneix P, Harvey T, Atienza P. Anal sphincter injury after forceps delivery: myth or reality? Diseases of the Colon & Rectum 2004;47: 24-34.

[11] Gudmundsson S, Henningsson AC, Lindqvist P. Correlation of birth injury with material height and birthweight. British Journal of Obstetrics and Gynaecology 2005;112(6): 764-7.

[12] Fernando R, Sultan AH, Kettle C, Thakar R, Radley S. Methods of repair for obstetric anal sphincter injury. Cochrane Database Systematic Reviews 2006;19: 3-CD002866.

[13] Choi JS, Wexner SD, Nam YS, Mavrantonis C, Salum M R, Yamaguchi T Weiss EG, Nogueras JJ, Yu CF. Intraobserver and interobserver measurements of the anorectal angle and perineal descent in defecography. Diseases of the Colon & Rectum 2000; vol 43,(8): 1121-6.

[14] Devine JB, Ostergard DR, Noblett KL. Long term complications of the second stage of labor. Obstetrics & Gynecology 1993;44(6): 119-21.

[15] Gregory WT, Lou JS, Stuyvesant A, Clark AL. Quantitative electromyography of anal sphincter after uncomplicated vaginal delivery. Obstetrics & Gynecology 2004;104: 327-35.

[16] Allen RE, Hosker GL, Smith ARB, Warrell DW. Pelvic floor damage and childbirth: a neurophysiological study. British Journal of Obstetrics and Gynaecology 1990;97: 770-9.

[17] Casey BM, Schaffer JI, Steven L, Bloom SL, Heartwell SF, McIntire DD. Obstetric antecedents for postpartum pelvic floor dysfunction. American Journal of Obstetrics and Gynaecology 2005;192: 1655-62.

[18] Jünemann K, Thüroff J. Innervation. In: Schüssler B, Laycock J, Norton P, Stanton S (eds.) Pelvic floor re-education. Principles and practice. London, Berlin, Heidelberg, New York, Paris, Tokyo, Hong Kong, Barcelona, Budapest: Springer-Verlag, 1994. p22-7.

[19] Snooks SS, Swash M, Henry MM, Setchell M. Risk Factors in childbirth causing damage to pelvic floor innervations. British Journal of Surgery 1985;72: 15-7.

[20] Schouten WR, Briel JW, Auwerda JJA. Relationship between anal pressure and anodermal blood flow. The vascular pathogenesis of anal fissures. Diseases of the Colon & Rectum 1994;37: 664-9.

[21] Hill K, Fanning S, Fennerty MB, Faigel DO. Endoanal ultrasound compared to anorectalmanometry for the evaluation of fecal incontinence: a study of the effect these tests have on clinical outcome. Digestive Diseases & Sciences 2006;51(2): 235-40.

[22] Argov S, Levandovsky O. Open lateral sphincterotomy is still the best treatment for chronic anal fissure. American Journal of Surgery 2000;179(3): 201-2.

[23] Kastinelos P, Papaziogas B, Koutelidakis I, Paroutoglou G, Dimiropoulos S,Souparis A, Atmatzidis K. Topical 0,5% nifedipine vs lateral internal sphincterotomy for the

treatment of chronic anal fissurae: long- term follow-up. The International Journal of Colorectal Disease 2006;21: 179-83.

[24] Richard CS, Gregoire R, Plewes EA, Silverman R, Burul C, Buie D, Reznick R, Ross T, Burnstein M, O'Connor BI, Mukraj D, McLeod RS. Internal sphincterotomy is superior to nitroglycerin in the treatment of chronic anal fissurae: results of a randomized, controlled trial by the Canadian Colorectal Surgical Trials Group. Diseases of the Colon & Rectum 2000;43: 1048-57.

[25] Ouaïssi M, Giger U, Sielezneff I, Yawovi KA, Pamela A, Pirro N, Sastre B.Mucosal advancement flap anoplasty for chronic anal fissure resistant to conservative therapy. World Journal of Surgery 2011;35(4): 900-4.

[26] Patel SD, Oxenham T, Praveen BV. Medium-term results of anal advancement flap compared with lateral sphincterotomy for the treatment of anal fissurae. The International Journal of Colorectal Disease; 26(9): 1211-4.

[27] Lasheen AE, Morsy MM, Fiad AA. Segmental internal sphincterotomy - a new technique for treatment of chronic anal fissure. Journal of Gastrointestinal Surgery 2011;15: 2271-4.

[28] Sohn N, Eisenberg MM, Weinstein MA, Lugo RN, Ader J. Precise anorectal sphincter dilatation - its role in the therapy of anal fissures. Diseases of the Colon & Rectum 1992;35 (4): 322-7.

[29] Renzi A. Clinical, manometric and ultrasonographic results of pneumatic balloon dilatation vs lateral internal sphincterotomy for chronic anal fissurae: a prospective, randomized controlled trial. Diseases of the Colon & Rectum 2008;51 (1): 121-7.

[30] van der Hagen SJ, Baeten CG, Soeters PB, van Gemert WG. Long-term outcome following mucosal advancement flap for high perianal fistulas and fistulotomy for low perianal fistulas: recurrent perianal fistulas: failure of treatment or recurrent patient disease? The International Journal of Colorectal Disease 2006;21: 784–90.

[31] Bokhari S,Lindsey I. Incontinence following sphincter division for treatment of anal fistula. The International Journal of Colorectal Disease 2010;12: 135-9.

[32] Perez F, Arroyo A, Serrano P et al. Fistulotomy with primary sphincter reconstruction in the management of complex fistula-in-ano: prospective study of clinical and manometric results. The Journal of the American College of Surgeons 2005;200: 897-903.

[33] Gemsenjager E. Results with a new therapy concept in anal fistula:suture of the anal sphincter. Schweizerische Medizinische Wochenschrift 1996;126: 2021-5.

[34] Jordan J, Roig JV, Garcia-Amengol J García-Granero E, Solana A, Lledó S.Risk Factors for reccurence and incontinence after anal fistula surgery. The International Journal of Colorectal Disease 2010;12: 254-60.

[35] Garg P, Song J, Bhatia A, Kalia H, Menon GR. The efficacy of anal fistula plug in fistula in ano. A systematic reviews of Colorectal Disease 2010;12: 965-70.

[36] Soltani A, Kaiser AM. Endorectal advancement flap for cryptoglandular or Crohn's fistula-in-ano. Diseases of the Colon & Rectum 2010;53: 486-95.

[37] Ritchie RD, Sackier JM, Hodde JP. Incontinence rates after cutting seton treatment for anal fistula. The International Journal of Colorectal Disease 2009;11: 564-71

[38] Vial M, Pares D, Pera M, Grande L. Fecal incontinence after seton treatment for anal fistulae with and without surgical division of internal anal sphincter: a systematic review. The International Journal of Colorectal Disease 2010;12: 172-8.

[39] Jorge JMN, Wexner SD. Etiology and management of fecal incontinence. Dis Colon Rectum 1993; 36, 77-97.

[40] Rockwood TH, Church JM, Fleshman JW, Kane RL, Mavrantonis C, Thorson AG, Wexner SD, Bliss D, Lowry AC. Fecal incontinence quality of life scale. Diseases of the Colon & Rectum 2000;vol 43(1): 9-16.

[41] Vaizey CJ, Kamm MA. Prospective assessment of the clinical value of anorectal investigations. Digestion 2000;61: 207-14.

[42] Pescatori M, Maria G, Anastazio G, Rinallo G. Anal manometry improves the outcome of surgery for fistula-in-ano. Diseases of the Colon & Rectum 1989;32(7): 588-592.

[43] Merletti R, Bottin A, Cescon C,Farina D, Gazzon M, Martina S,Mestin L, Pozzo M, Rainoldi A, Enck P. Multichannel surface EMG for the non-invasive assesment of the anal sphincter muscle. Digestion 2004;69 (2): 112-22.

[44] Fernardo RJ, Sultan AH. Risk factors and management of obstetric perineal injury. Current Obstetrics & Gynaecology 2004;14: 320-6.

Chapter 4

A Novel Concept on the Patho-Physiology of Defecation and Fecal Incontinence (FI) in Women – Moreover, Its Reconstructive Surgery

Abdel Karim M. El Hemaly, Laila A.E.S. Mousa, Ibrahim M. Kandil, Magdy S. Al Sayed, Mohammad Abdel Zaher, Magdi S.A. Soliman and Ahmad G. Serour

Additional information is available at the end of the chapter

1. Introduction

We put forward a new concept explaining the physiology of defecation and the anatomy of the internal anal sphincter (IAS). We explain the important role that the IAS plays in the control of defecation and fecal continence. Our aim is to explain the physiology of defection, factors that control fecal continence and causes of fecal incontinence in women together with the importance and the structure of the internal anal sphincter (IAS) and how it maintains fecal continence. The harmony between the central nervous system (CNS), the autonomic nervous system, the integrity of the anal sphincters and the muscles of the body are essential for keeping fecal continence. Traumatic injury can occur during childbirth affecting the anal sphincters and causing fecal incontinence (FI). Difficult vaginal deliveries can lead to more than one lesion at the same time. Simultaneous stress urinary incontinence (SUI), vaginal prolapse and fecal incontinence (FI) arise as a sequel to the cumulative trauma of recurrent frequent vaginal deliveries.

We will describe a novel technique for the surgical repair of vaginal wall prolapse, SUI and fecal incontinence.

Fecal Continence depends on a closed and empty anal canal, which in turn depends on four main factors:

1. The integrity of the two anal sphincters: (the internal anal sphincter (IAS) and the external anal sphincter (EAS); both anal sphincters must be intact with healthy and strong walls. Intact healthy vascular and nerve supply are important factors for anal sphincter function.
2. An acquired high alpha-sympathetic tone at the IAS that keeps the anal canal closed and empty at all times until there is a desire and/ or a need to pass flatus &/ or stool and under suitable social circumstances. The high alpha-sympathetic tone is gained by learning and training in early childhood.
3. Healthy and strong pelvic floor muscles, including the levator ani, that maintain the angle between the rectum and the anal canal.
4. Synchronization and synergistic actions between the central nervous system (CNS), the autonomic nervous system, peripheral somatic nerves, the muscles and the anal sphincters.

The closed and empty anal canal has a high anal pressure that is much higher than rectal pressure; rectal pressure reflects the abdominal pressure.

We put forward a novel concept on the patho-physiology of defecation (1,2,3,4) (figure 1).

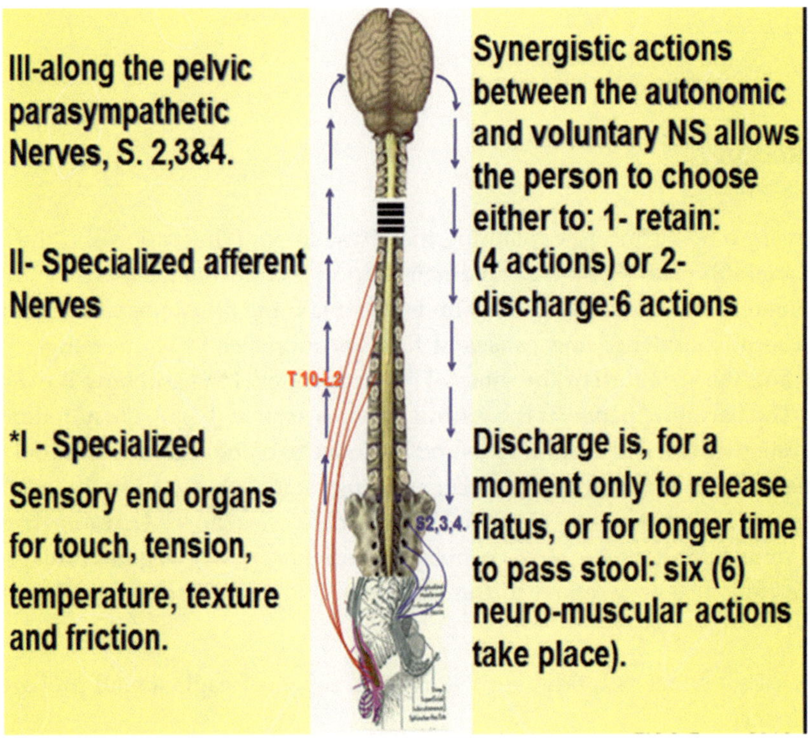

Figure 1. Physiology of defecation

Diagram that explains the steps that take place sequentially during defecation.

2. Defecation in infancy and early childhood, before training

Activation of stretch receptors in the rectum trigger impulses conveying rectal fullness which travel along the pelvic Parasympathetic (S2, 3 and 4) to the spinal cord sacral centers and lead to:

1. Reflex contraction of the rectal muscles.
2. Opening of the anal canal and relaxation of the external anal sphincter (EAS) allowing defection to occur.

Mothers start to teach their children from the age of about two to three years how to control themselves and hold on until favorable social circumstances allow defecation.

3. Gaining control of defecation

Gaining control is achieved by maintaining high alpha-sympathetic tone in the IAS keeping it contracted and the anal canal closed and empty at all times and until an appropriate place and time are available. On rectal distension, stretch receptors are stimulated. The sensation of rectal distension travels along the pelvic parasympathetic nerves to S 2, 3 and 4 to the sacral spinal cord centers. The ano-rectal junction contains specialized sensory end organs for tension, temperature, texture, touch and friction. Specialized afferent nerves sub serve these organized nerve endings. Controlled by the central nervous system (CNS), an intact sampling reflex allows the individual to choose whether to:

a. Retain the rectal contents or,
b. Discharge the contents whether flatus and/ or stool.

Dependent on the available social circumstances, and once maturational control of continence has been achieved, if the woman chooses to retain rectal contents until a later time when social circumstances are more favourable, then she will:

1. Increase acquired high alpha-sympathetic tone at the IAS, ensuring its contraction and closure of the anal canal.
2. Augment the contraction of the EAS, which is a voluntary muscle, innervated with somatic nerve supply.
3. Increase the contraction of the levator ani muscles to exaggerate the angle between the rectum and anal canal.
4. Inhibit pelvic parasympathetic activity to the colon and the rectum preventing their muscular contractions.

Discharge of the rectal contents occurs by relaxation of both anal sphincters (IAS & EAS) and the pelvic floor muscles, for a moment only to pass flatus, or for a longer time to release stool.

When, an appropriate time and place are available and there is a desire to evacuate, under the control of the high CNS centers, through synergistic synchronized nervous actions between the autonomic, and the voluntary nervous systems, six neuromuscular actions will occur:

1. The woman will lower the acquired high alpha-sympathetic tone at the IAS relaxing it, opening the anal canal.
2. Through the voluntary NS, she will relax the pelvic floor muscles thus annulling the ano-rectal angle, to bring the anal canal and the rectum on one axis. She does so through relaxing the pelvic floor muscles.
3. Through the voluntary NS, she will also relax the EAS, which is a skeletal muscle innervated by the pudendal nerve. Then two synergistic synchronized actions between the voluntary and autonomic nervous system will occur.
4. The abdominal muscles and the diaphragm contract to increase the intra-abdominal pressure thus forcing the feces through the anal canal (The voluntary nervous system controls this action).
5. The smooth muscles of the distal colon and rectum contract; propelling the feces into the anal canal then to outside, (The autonomic nervous system does this action).
6. Subsequently, there will be sequential contractions of the three parts of the EAS: the deep, then the superficial then the subcutaneous parts that will squeeze the anal canal propelling any residual contents and emptying the anal canal completely.

Fecal incontinence means involuntary escape of flatus, mucus and/ or stool. Fecal incontinence (FI) is one of the most distressing conditions, psychologically and socially, in any individual. It can lead to depression, social isolation, loss of self-esteem, loss of self-confidence and poor quality of life (QOL).

Causes of FI include (5-17):

a. Anal Sphincter damage: Traumatic injury to the anal sphincter, its nerve or blood supply, can lead to FI. Commonest causes are:
    1. Childbirth trauma,
    2. Trauma during and after surgery e.g. during performing surgical operation for piles; surgery for a pelvic or perineal tumor.
    3. Traumatic injury caused by exposure to irradiation.
    4. Damage of the nervous system.
b. Pelvic floor dysfunction:
    1. Rectocele,
    2. Rectal prolapse,
    3. Generalized weakness and sagging of the pelvic floor.

c. Pelvic floor neuromuscular damage e.g. decreased perception of rectal sensations, decrease anal canal pressure, decreased squeeze pressure of the anal canal & impaired anal sensation.

d. Constipation: Constipation is a common cause of fecal incontinence (it is similar to retention with overflow in urinary incontinence, UI). Constipation causes prolonged muscle and nerve stretching and leads to weakness of the intestinal muscles and nerves resulting in fecal incontinence.

e. Diarrhea: Diarrhea, (similar to urge and urge incontinence in UI; overactive bladder in urinary incontinence) loose stool is more difficult to control than solid stool.

Diarrhea can be:

1. Acute: e.g. G.I. infections, food poisoning.

2. Chronic: e.g. ulcerative colitis, Crohn's disease, diverticulitis or neoplasm; gastrectomy, vagotomy; malabsorption; thyrotoxicosis. When the cause of diarrhea is temporary such as G.I. infections or food reactions, incontinence tends to last for a short period.

f. Nerve damage: damage to the autonomic, voluntary nervous systems or to the CNS can lead to FI.

The sensation of rectal distension travels along the parasympathetic system to S 2, 3& 4. Damage to the sensory nerves &/or the motor nerves; or to the CNS can cause FI. If the damage affects the sensory nerves, detection of stool in the rectum is disabled, and one will not feel the need to defecate until it is too late.

Causes of nerve damage include:

1. Childbirth trauma,

2. Long-term constipation,

3. Cerebral vascular accident, stroke,

Neuropathy result of diseases such as diabetes mellitus, systemic lupus erthrymatosis (SLE) and disseminated sclerosis (DS).

g. Loss of storage capacity of the rectum:

Normally, the rectum stretches to hold stool until it is voluntarily discharged. However, rectal surgery, radiation treatment, and inflammatory bowel disease can cause scarring of the rectal wall. The rectal walls are unable to stretch as much and are unable to accommodate as much stool. Inflammatory bowel disease also can make rectal walls very irritated and thereby unable to keep stool

h. Other causes:

Fecal incontinence can have other causes including one or a combination of the following:

1. Congenital causes: In cases of imperforate anus, partial or complete lack of the sphincter mechanism (rare).
2. Patulous anus is associated with mental retardation.
3. Malabsorption conditions e.g. cystic fibrosis; drugs; and indigestible dietary fats that interfere with the intestinal absorption will lead to FI.
4. Lateral internal sphincterotomy (surgery for anal fissures); and surgery for high fistula-in-ano.
5. Seizures and fits.
6. Perineal resection of the rectum for carcinoma.

A major cause of fecal incontinence in young healthy women is anal sphincter damage during vaginal delivery, which occurs in as many as 18% in the USA. Studies from other countries indicate 5-20% of women report incontinence of stool 3-6 months after sphincter tear (EAS), and 29-53% of women report incontinence of flatus, despite having the tear repaired at delivery (5).

Surgical repair of the torn EAS is by suturing end-to-end the torn edges of the EAS; or suturing after overlapping the torn edges. All published reports of the results of overlapping technique have shown significant improvements in symptoms of FI, with 60-80% achieving continence (6). It is also clear, however, that fecal control deteriorates over time with only 50% of the initial successful outcomes having improved continence at five years (7). Poor understanding of perineal anatomy and inadequate training in repair techniques are possible reasons for the high incidence of persistent symptoms (6,7). In addition, this can explain why repair of the EAS in cases of complete perineal tear whether by end-to-end or overlapping techniques does not lead to complete continence (7).

The problem is that the role of the Internal Anal Sphincter (IAS) in defecation and FI is not quite clear.

We will describe the IAS in a novel way and its important role in maintaining fecal continence and defecation (1, 2, 33), (figure 2).

The IAS is a collagen-muscle tissue cylinder that surrounds the anal canal, and is in turn surrounded externally in its lower part by the EAS. Its nerve supply is from the alpha-sympathetic nerves coming through the thoracolumbar alpha-sympathetic nerves, from the hypogastric plexus (T10-L2). The collagen constitutes the firm frame (chassis) of the IAS, while the muscle is the mover of the sphincter in response to nerve stimulus. Its functions are:

1. On contraction, to keep the anal canal closed and empty with high anal pressure.
2. On relaxation, to open the anal canal to allow passage of flatus and/ or stool.

An intact and strong IAS, through the acquired high alpha-sympathetic tone that maintains its contraction, keeps the anal canal closed and empty with high anal pressure, much higher than the rectal pressure.

The IAS is in close relation to the posterior vaginal wall, which stretches very much during labor. Prolonged labor, difficult, multiple frequent labors cause overstretching of the posterior vaginal wall, leading to flabbiness of the vagina with subsequent falling down of the redundant vaginal wall, posterior vaginal wall prolapse (rectocele). The redundancy of the vaginal wall is the result of rupture of its collagenous sheet (the vaginal firm frame). The rupture will affect and damage the intimately related IAS with subsequent FI. The rupture in the IAS affects the collagen layer (the collagen frame). Damage of the IAS causes dilation of the anal canal. Open and dilated anal canal with a lowered pressure allows the rectal contents to enter the open anal canal with subsequent fecal incontinence. Therefore, we can more correctly say that the first cause of FI is anal sphincter damage, with traumatic injury to one and/or both anal sphincters, IAS, EAS (figures: 3 to 15).

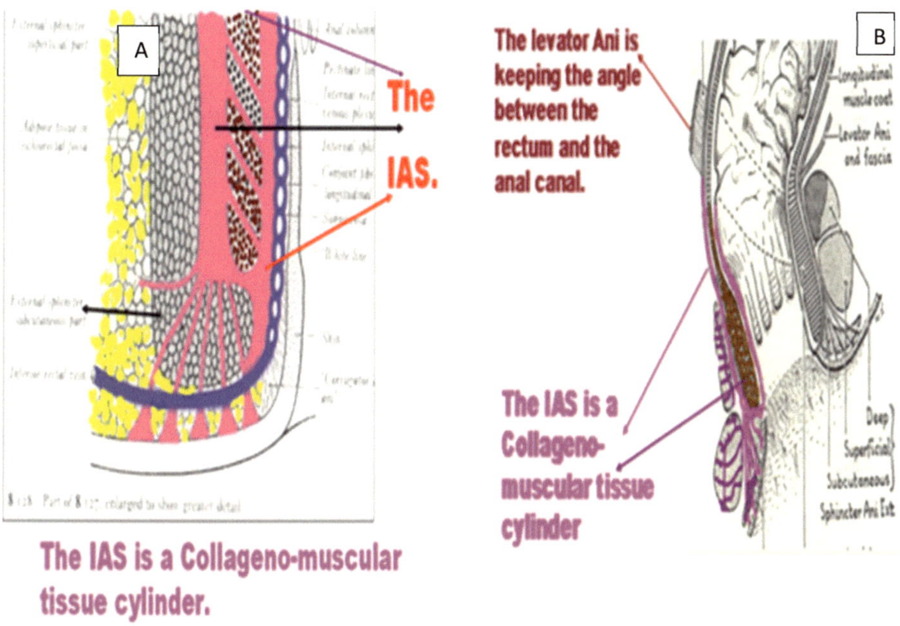

(A)- Gray's Anatomy: Roger Warwick and Peter L. Williams (editors), 35th edition; Longman Group Ltd, 1973; anal musculature, 1293. Colors by author.

(B)- Clinical Anatomy: A Revision and Applied Anatomy for Clinical Students, fifth edition, Harold Ellis (editor); Blackwell Scientific Publications, 1972; 80. Colors by author.

Figure 2. The anatomy of the internal anal sphincter (IAS). The IAS, according to the new description, is a cylinder of collagen-muscle tissue that surrounds the anal canal. The external anal sphincter (EAS), with its three sections surrounds the IAS.

Three dimension ultrasound (3DUS) images of the rectum and anal canal with torn IAS in patients with fecal incontinence (FI).

FI is the main complaint in posterior vaginal wall prolapse (rectocele). Concomitant troubles, which commonly occur, are vaginal prolapse (anterior and posterior), stress urinary incontinence (SUI) and FI (1) (Figures: 13, 14 &15). The internal urethral sphincter (IUS) is in close contact to the anterior vaginal wall and will be involved in the childbirth trauma with subsequent SUI and anterior vaginal wall prolapse.

Childbirth trauma is the major cause of damage, but aging, hormone deficiency (menopause) and degeneration from chronic and/or repeated infections causing collagen degeneration and atrophy can add to the weakness of the internal urethral sphincter (IUS), IAS and the vagina.

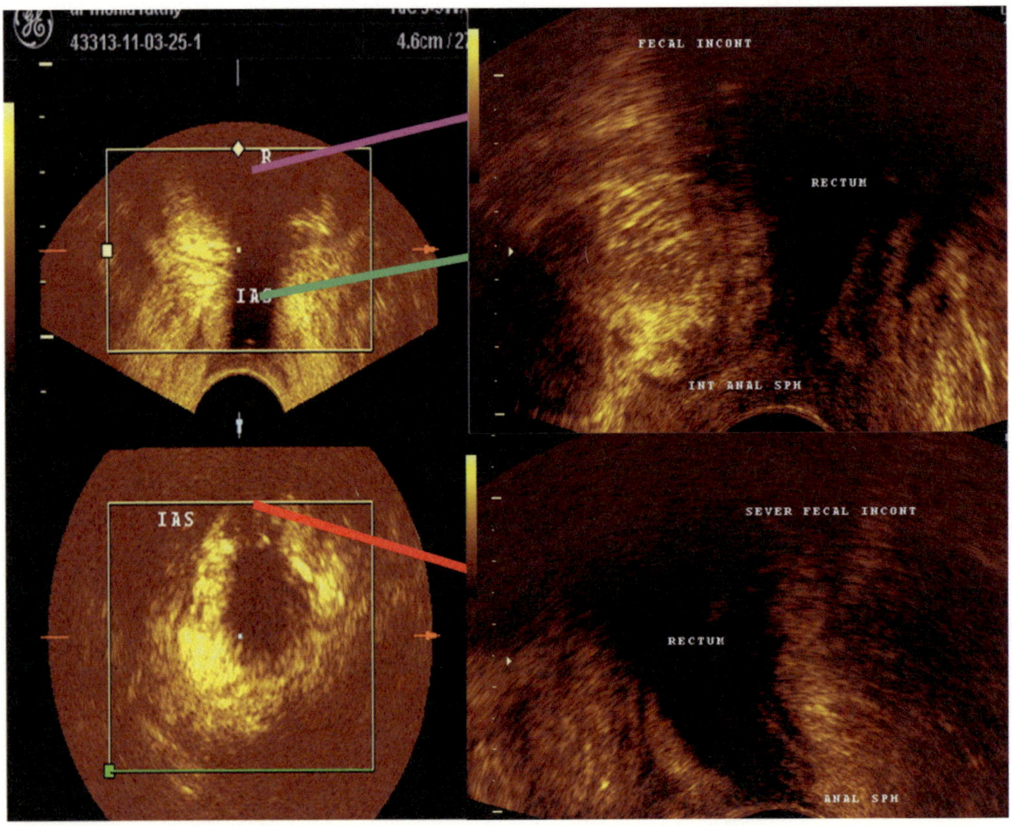

Figure 3. MRI images of a continent patient, (A), with an intact internal urethral sphincter (IUS), an intact IAS with a closed and empty anal canal. In addition, the vagina is standing up and not prolapsed. In contrast, patient, (B) suffers from urinary incontinence, FI and vaginal prolapse as demonstrated by torn IUS, IAS and vagina.

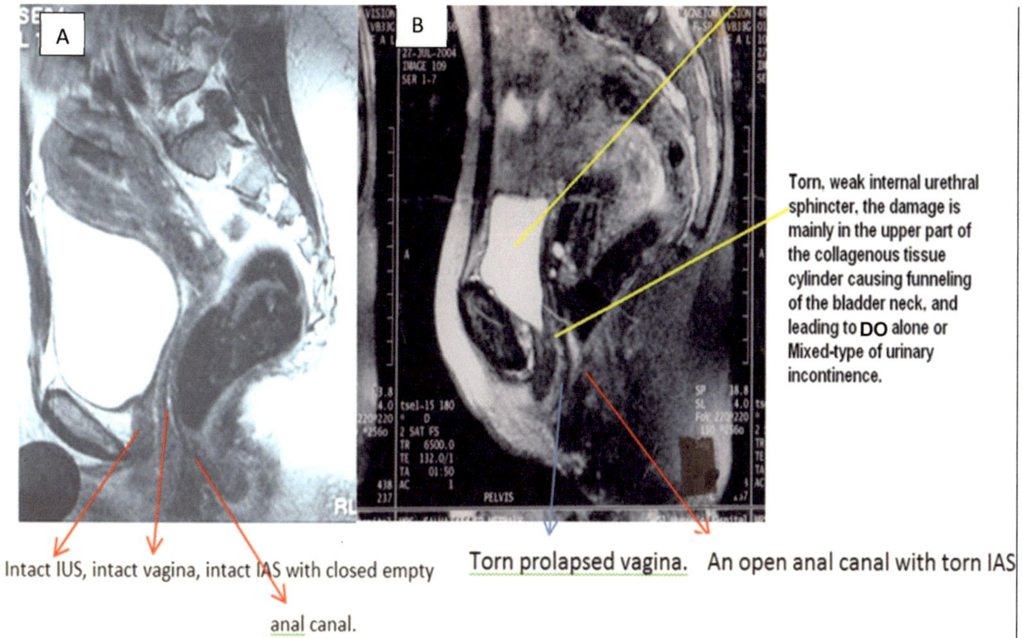

Figure 4. MRI images of a patient who suffers from SUI and FI. The IUS is torn especially in its upper part with funneling of the bladder neck, and torn IAS with an open anal canal.

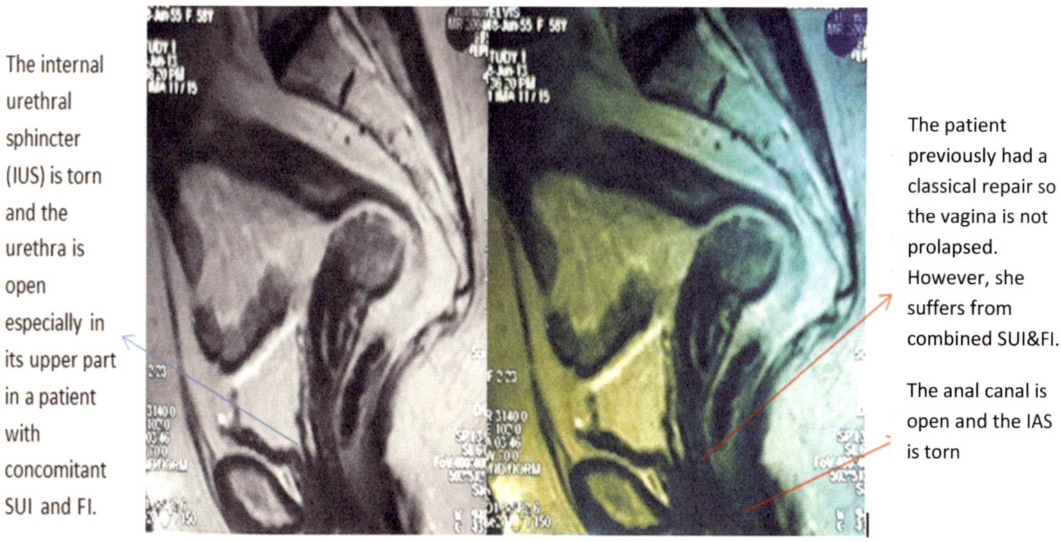

Figure 5. MRI images of a patient who suffers from SUI and FI. The IUS is torn especially in its upper part with funneling of the bladder neck, and torn IAS with an open anal canal.

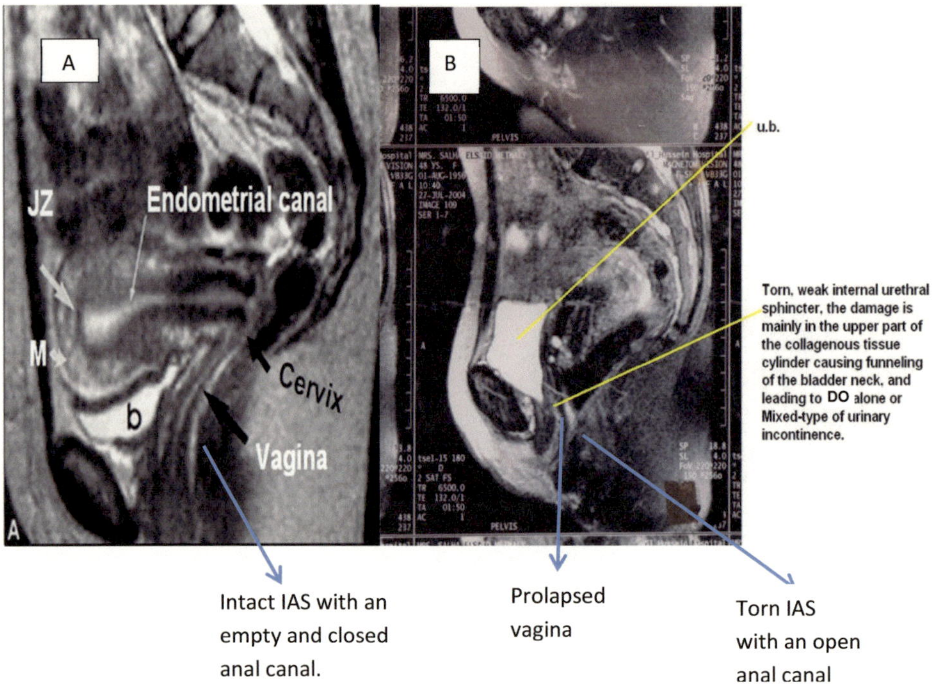

Figure 6. MRI images of a normal continent woman (A) with intact IUS, IAS with a closed empty anal canal and normal non-prolapsing vagina. Image (B) is of an incontinent patient with torn IUS and torn IAS and prolapsed vagina.

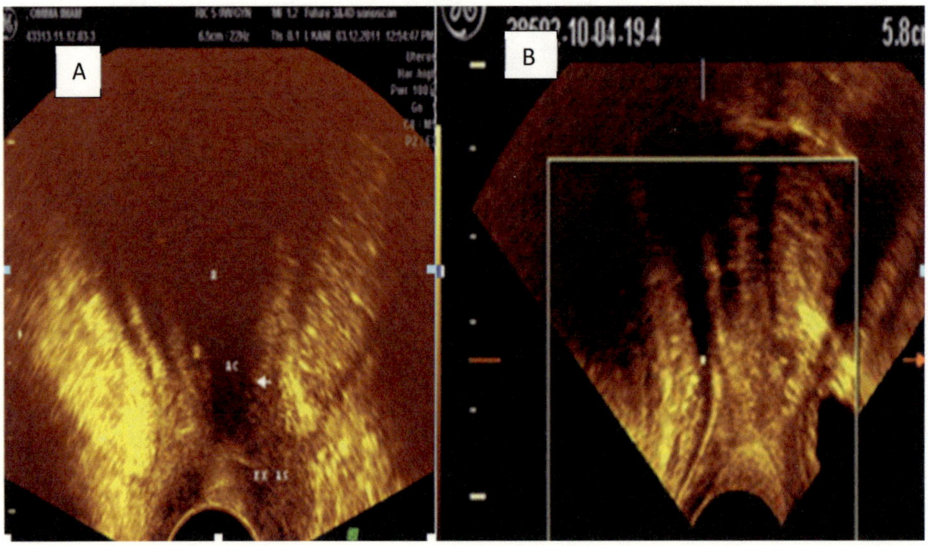

Figure 7. Images with 3DUS of the rectum and anal canal in normal continent woman (B) with healthy, intact IAS and a closed empty anal canal. In contrast, in (A) the IAS is torn leading to a widely open anal canal in a patient with FI.

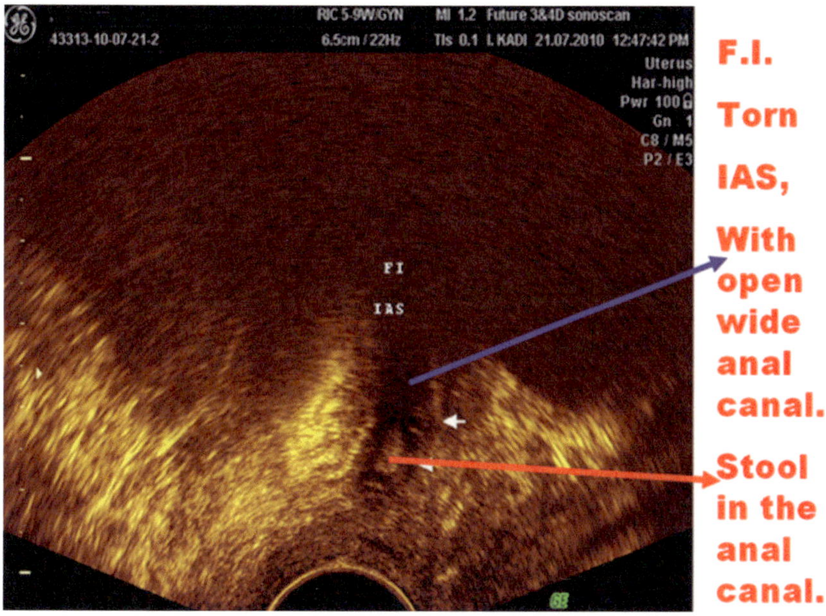

Figure 8. An image with 3DUS of a patient with FI that shows torn IAS, and an open anal canal with a piece of stool in the anal canal.

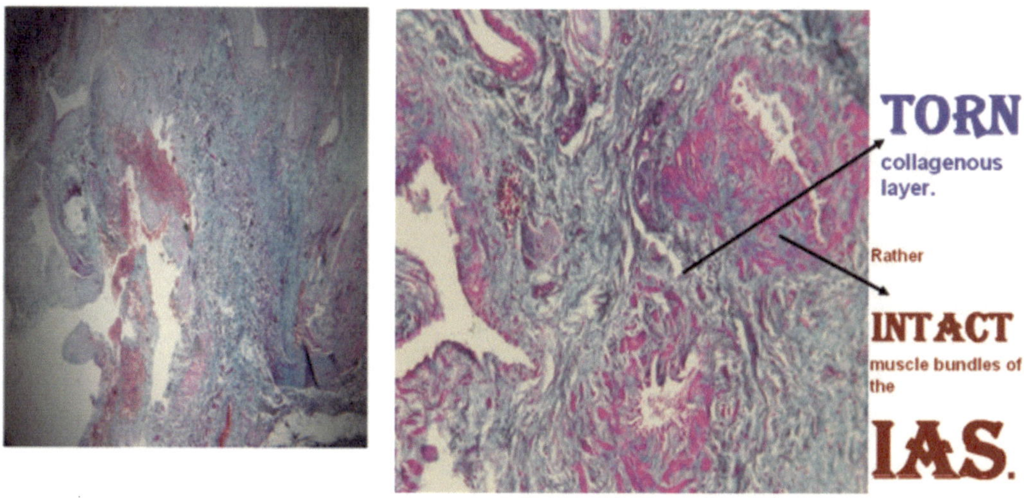

Figure 9. Histopathology of a surgical specimen of the IAS stained with Masson trichrome acetate, showing a torn collagen sheet with relative healthy muscle bundles.

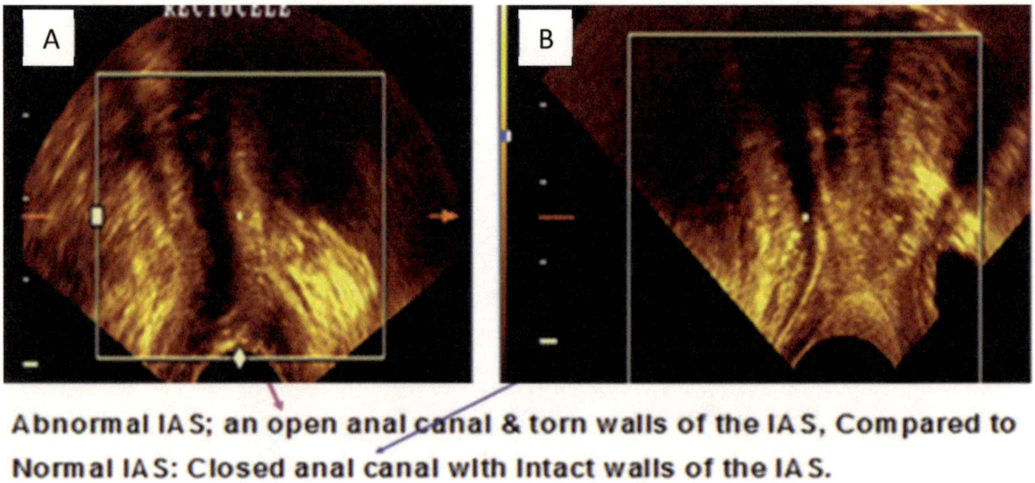

Figure 10. Images with 3DUS of the rectum and anal canal in a normal continent woman (B) with a healthy, intact IAS and a closed empty anal canal. In contrast, in (A) the IAS is torn leading to a widely open anal canal in a patient with FI.

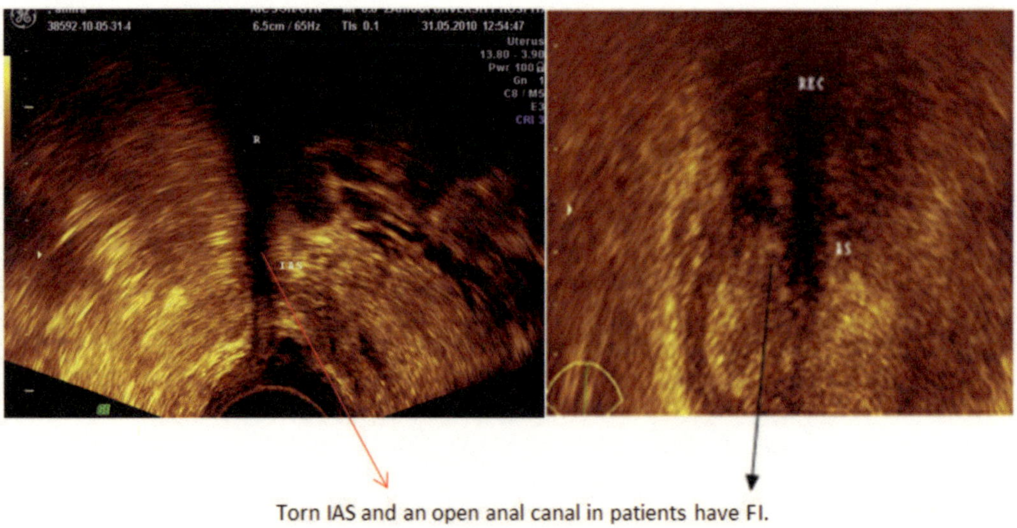

Figure 11. Images with 3DUS of patients with FI. The IAS is torn and the anal canal is open.

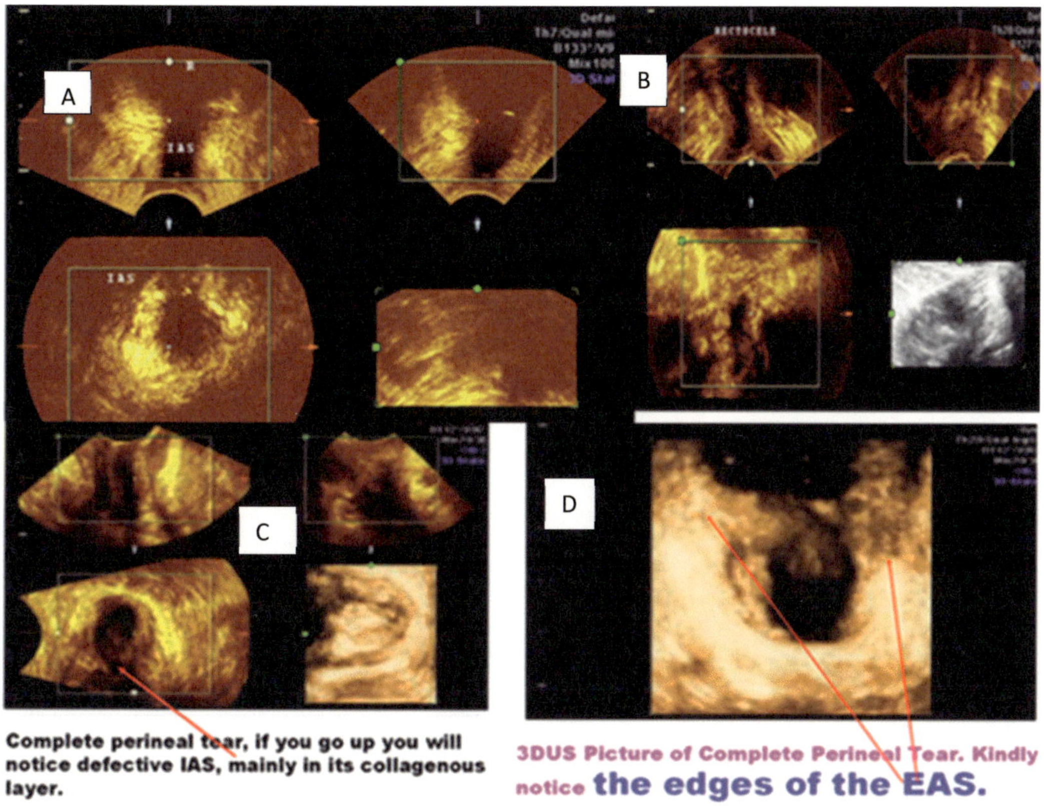

Figure 12. Images with 3DUS of the rectum and anal canal in patients with FI. Images in C & D are of a complete perineal tear (fourth degree). The external anal sphincter is torn and appears as a horseshoe; in addition, the internal anal sphincter is torn as well. Images in A and B are of the internal anal sphincter, which is torn leading to an open dilated anal canal. The IAS in this image also appears like a horseshoe.

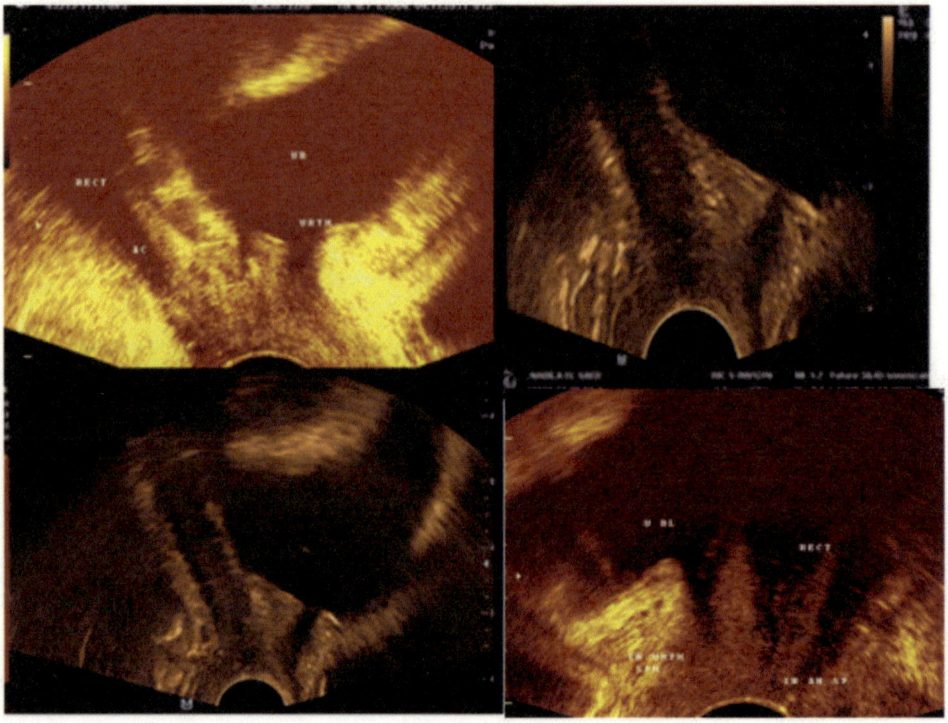

Figure 13. images of patients who suffer from pelvic organ dysfunction with SUI, FI and vaginal prolapse simultaneously. The images show torn IUS and IAS.

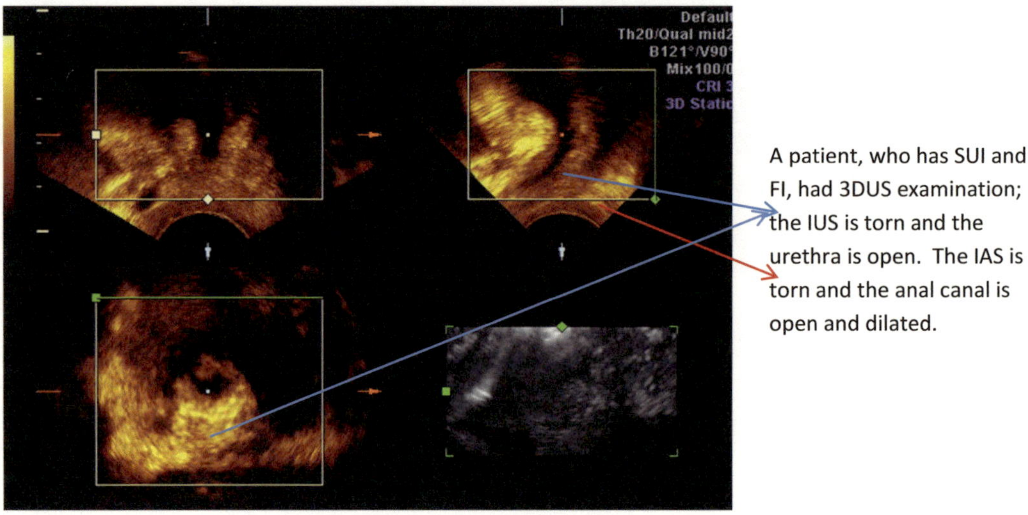

Figure 14. images which show concomitant torn IUS and IAS in a patient who suffers pelvic floor dysfunction

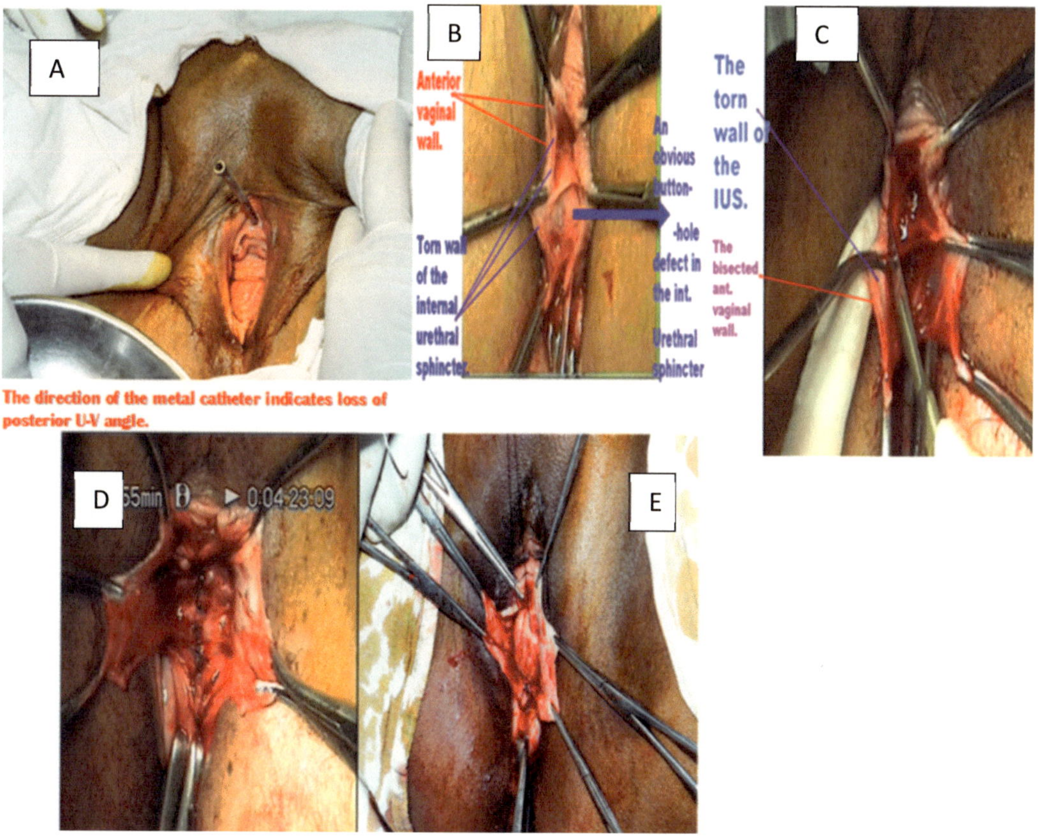

Figure 15. Surgical photos of a patient with anterior vaginal wall prolapse, posterior vaginal wall prolapse, SUI, and FI. The metal catheter is directed forward and upward (A), which means loss of posterior urethro-vesical angle. We dissect the IUS from the anterior vaginal wall (B&C) and mended the torn IUS with simple interrupted sutures (D&E).

In addition, anal intercourse can cause traumatic damage of the IAS with subsequent FI (1, 2 & 3).

4. Diagnosis

In addition to the clinical history and examination, imaging with three-dimension ultrasound (3DUS) and magnetic resonance (MRI) is an essential tool in the management of cases of FI. Typically, it shows an open anal canal with torn IAS. It may also reveal an open urethra and torn IUS with concomitant SUI and vaginal prolapse (figures: 3, 4, 5, 6, 7, 8, 10, 11, 12, 13 & 14). Histopathological examination of a torn piece of the IAS confirm that the rupture mainly affects the collagen frame of the IAS (figure 9).

5. Reconstructive surgery (figures: 15, 16, 17, 18 & 19)

In conclusion, a major cause of FI in young patients is torn IAS. We have developed an operative procedure to expose and mend the torn edges of the IAS. Since there is usually concomitant vaginal prolapse and SUI, we try to correct these concurrently as part of this new operation.

"Urethro-Ano-Vaginoplasty" "Al Azhar repair operation"

The operation consists of Anterior and Posterior sections.

In the Anterior section, we correct the SUI and the anterior vaginal wall descent through the following steps: (Figures: 15 & 16).

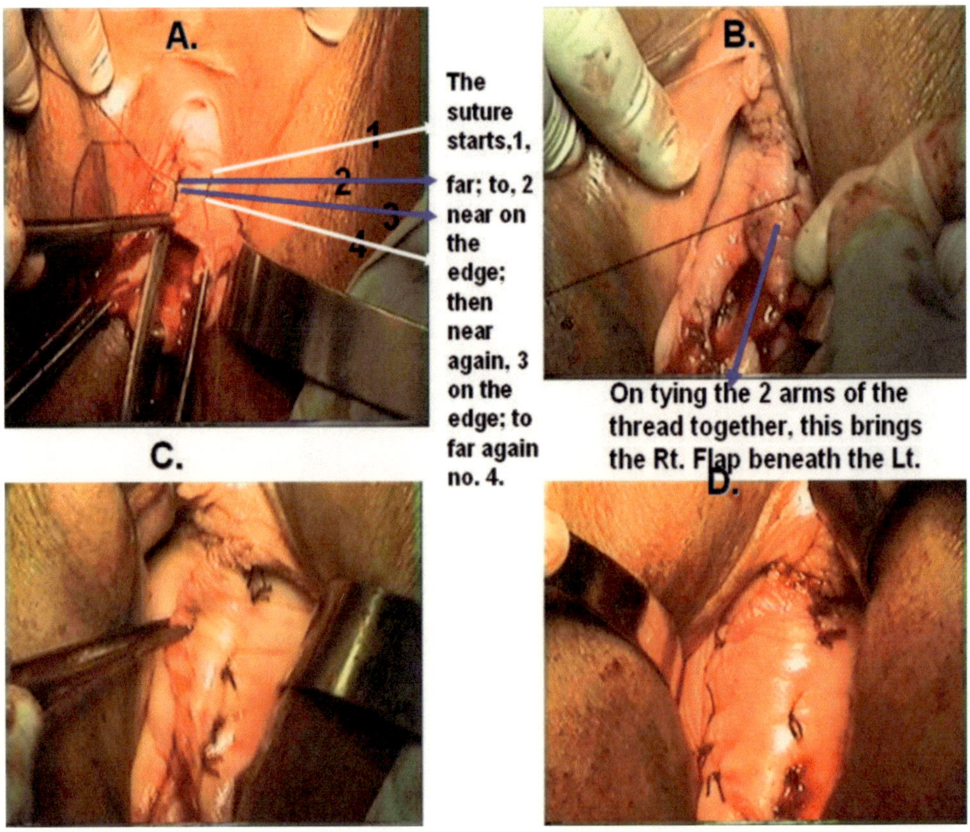

Figure 16. After mending the IUS, we do overlapped the two vaginal flaps as seen in the photos. We bring the right vaginal flap underneath the left vaginal flap with this novel dragging suture as seen in (A) and (B), repeating it 4-6 times. Then we suture the free edge of the left vaginal flap as far laterally in the vagina on the right as seen in C& D. Thus, we strengthen the anterior vaginal wall and add extra strength to the mended IUS.

We grasp the cervix with two pairs of cervical volsela. We inject about 10-20 ml. normal saline with adrenaline (2 per 200 thousand concentration}, beneath the vaginal wall to act as a hydro dissection and vasoconstrictor. This separates the anterior vaginal wall from the posterior wall of the IUS. We make a 2-4 cm transverse incision about three cm above the external cervical os. With a pair of dissecting scissors, we separate the anterior vaginal wall from the IUS. We cut the anterior vaginal wall longitudinally from the transverse cut all the way, "down", to the submeatal sulcus, which correspond to the perineal membrane. We grasp each vaginal flap with three pairs of Kocher's forceps. The defect in the IUS will be apparent and on each side, we can clearly see two clear edges. One edge is of the anterior vaginal wall and the other is the torn posterior wall of the IUS.

1. Expose the IUS (we dissect the IUS clear from the anterior vaginal wall).
2. Mend the torn posterior wall of the IUS by several (6-8) simple interrupted sutures using number 0 polyglycan thread, sutures (figure 15).
3. Strengthen the anterior vaginal wall by overlapping the two vaginal flaps, using a novel dragging sutures, dragging the right vaginal flap underneath the left vaginal flap. Then we suture the free edge of the left vaginal flap as far lateral on the right side of the vagina. This strengthens the anterior vaginal wall and decreases its width, also adding extra support to the mended IUS, and preserving the body collagen.

Posterior section (figures: 17, 18 & 19).

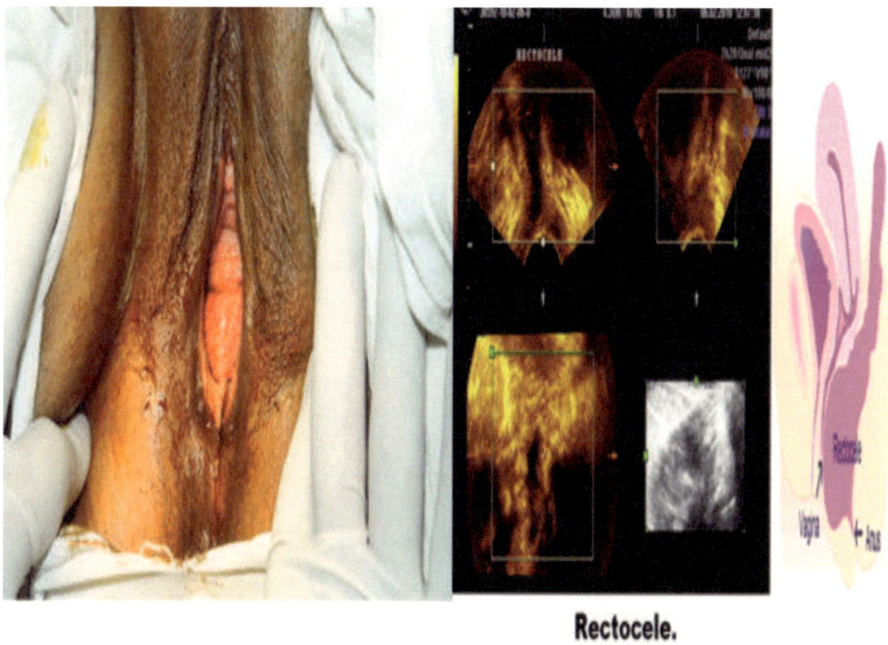

Figure 17. Image A clearly shows the posterior vaginal wall even without straining. This is visible with posterior vaginal wall prolapse. Image (B) is 3DUS showing rectocele of the same patient who suffers FI.

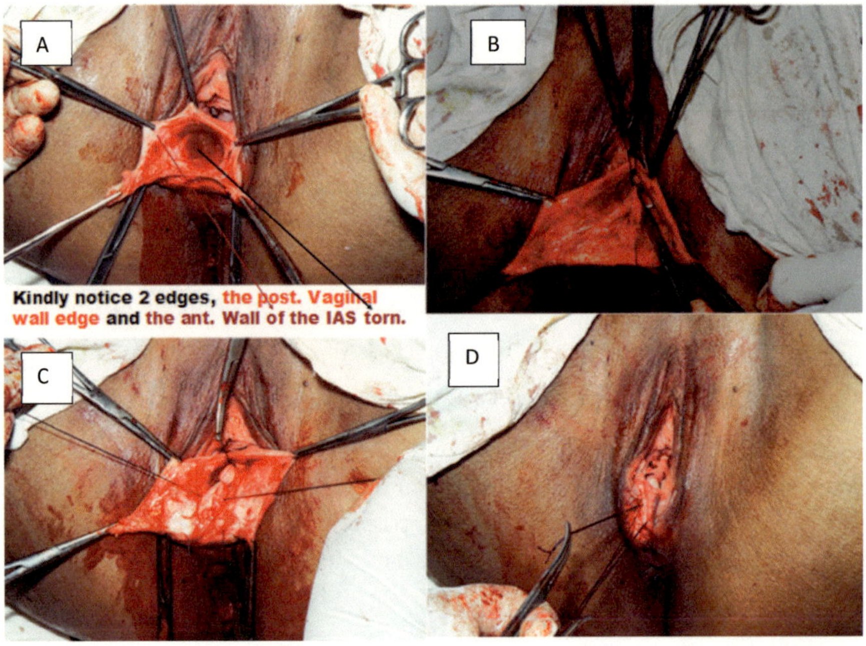

Figure 18. Surgical steps of posterior repair. We dissect the IAS from the posterior vaginal wall (A). We mend the sphincter (B&C), in addition, we approximate the two levator ani muscles by two stitches, but we do not tie them till we finish overlapping the posterior vaginal wall (D).

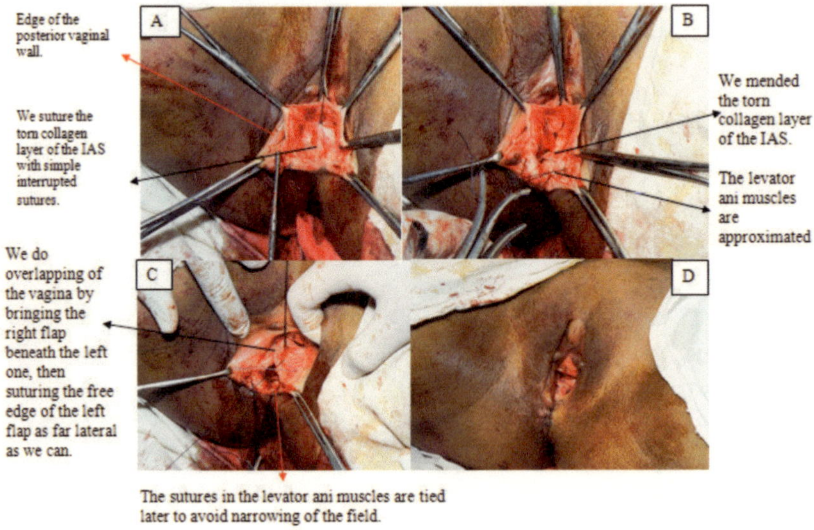

Figure 19. Images that show the steps taken to expose the torn IAS and mend it (A&B). We then overlapped the redundant posterior vaginal wall as is seen in (C). Next, we approximated the two levator ani muscles; and finally repaired the perineum as is seen in (D).

We hydro dissect between the posterior vaginal wall, the anal canal and the rectum; and in the perineum as described for the anterior section.

We make a V-shape incision at the line between the posterior vaginal wall and the perineal skin down to the perineum. Then we try to create a space between the posterior vaginal wall and the anal canal by sharp and blunt dissection. Next with a pair of dissecting scissors, we separate the posterior vaginal wall from the rectum and anal canal. Then we cut the posterior vaginal wall longitudinally in the midline to beyond the apex of the prolapse protrusion. We hold each vaginal flap with three pairs of Kocher's forceps. Two different edges can clearly be seen on each side, one is the vaginal edge, and the other is the anterior wall of the torn IAS.

1. We dissect the torn IAS clear from the posterior vaginal wall.
2. Mend the torn wall of the sphincter by serial interrupted simple sutures with number 0 polyglcan thread.
3. Approximate the two levator ani muscles.
4. Strengthen the posterior vaginal wall by overlapping the two vaginal flaps; thus, we also add extra support to the mended IAS and keeping the natural body collagen.
5. Repair the perineum.

We put a Foley's catheter and vagina pack for 24 hours.

List of abbreviations

3DUS: Three-Dimension Ultra Sound.

CNS: Central Nervous System.

EAS: External Anal Sphincter.

EAS: External Anal Sphincter.

EUS: External Urethral Sphincter.

FI: Fecal Incontinence.

GI: Gastro-Intestinal.

IAS: Internal Anal Sphincter.

IUS: Internal Urethral Sphincter

MRI: Magnetic Resonance Imaging.

NS: Nervous System.

QOL: Quality Of Life.

SUI: Stress Urinary Incontinence.

T10-L2: Thoracic 10 to Lumbar two.

UI: Urinary Incontinence.

Author details

Abdel Karim M. El Hemaly[1], Laila A.E.S. Mousa[1], Ibrahim M. Kandil[1], Magdy S. Al Sayed[2], Mohammad Abdel Zaher[1,3], Magdi S.A. Soliman[3] and Ahmad G. Serour[1]

*Address all correspondence to: profakhemaly@hotmail.com

1 Al Azhar University, Cairo, Egypt

2 University Hospital, Salman Bin Abdul Aziz University, K.S.A., Egypt

3 Salman Bin Abdul Aziz University, K.S.A., Egypt

References

[1] Abdel Karim M El Hemaly, Laila A Mousa, Asim Kurjak, Ibrahim M Kandil, Ahmad G Serour. Pelvic Floor Dysfunction, the Role of Imaging and Reconstructive Surgery, Donald School Journal of Ultrasound in Obstetrics and Gynecology, DSJUOG, January-March 2013;7(1):86-97

[2] Abdel Karim M. El Hemaly*, Ibrahim M. Kandil, Asim Kurjak, Laila A. S. Mousa, Hossam H. Kamel, Ahmad G. Serour. Ultrasound Assessment of the Internal Anal Sphincter in Women with Fecal Incontinence and Posterior Vaginal Wall Prolapse (Rectocele). Donald School Journal of Ultrasound in Obstetrics and Gynecology, DSJUOG, vol. 5, No 4, 330-42; October-December 2011.

[3] Abdel Karim M. El Hemaly*, Laila A. S. Mousa Ibrahim M. Kandil, Fatma S. El Sokkary, Ahmad G. Serour, Hossam Hussein. Fecal Incontinence, A Novel Concept: The Role of the internal Anal sphincter (IAS) in defecation and fecal incontinence. Gynaecologia et Perinatologia, Vol19, No 2; 79-85 April -June 2010.

[4] Abdel Karim M. El Hemaly*, Laila A. S. Mousa Ibrahim M. Kandil, Fatma S. El Sokkary, Ahmad G. Serour, Hossam Hussein. Surgical Treatment of Stress Urinary Incontinence, Fecal Incontinence and Vaginal Prolapse by A Novel Operation "Urethro-Ano-Vaginoplasty" Gynaecologia et Perinatologia, Vol19, No 3; 129-188 July-September 2010.

[5] Pinta TM, Kylanpaa ML, Salmi TK, et al. Primary sphincter repair: Are the results of the operation good enough? Dis Colon Rectum 2004; 47:18-23.

[6] France-Borello Diane, Kathryn L.Burgio, Holly E. Richter, Hallina Zycnski, Mary Pat Fitzgerald, William Whitehead, Paul Fine, Ingrid Nygaard, Victoria L. Handa, Anthony G. Vesco, Anne M. Wiber and Morton B. Brown; PhD, for the Pelvic Floor Disorders, Network, Fecal and Urinary incontinence in primiparous women. Obstet & Gynecol 2006; 108(4):863-72.

[7] Halverson AL, Hull TL. Long-term outcome of overlapping anal sphincter repair. Dis Colon Rectum 2002; 45:345-48.

[8] Sultan AH, Thakar R. Lower genital tract and anal sphincter trauma. Best Pract Res Clin Obstet Gyecol 2002; 16:99-115.

[9] Faltin DL, Boulvain M, Floris LA, et al. Diagnosis of anal sphincter tears to prevent fecal incontinence: a randomized controlled trial. Obstet Gynecol 2005;106(1): 6–13.

[10] Nichols CM, Ramakrishnan V, Gill EJ, et al. Anal incontinence in women with and those without pelvic floor disorders. Obstet Gynecol 2005; 106(6): 1266–71.

[11] Dietz HP, Lanzarone V. Levator trauma after vaginal delivery. Obstet Gynecol 2005;106(4):707–12.

[12] Jackson SL, Weber AM, Hull TL, et al. Fecal incontinence in women with urinary incontinence and pelvic organ prolapse. Obstet Gynecol 1997; 89(3):423–7.

[13] Mimura T, Kaminishi M, Kamm MA. Diagnostic evaluation of patients with faecal incontinence at a specialist institution. Dig Surg 2004; 21(3):235–41

[14] Kruger JA, Heap SW, Murphy BA, et al. Pelvic floor function in nulliparous women using three-dimensional ultrasound and magnetic resonance imaging. Obstet Gynecol 2008;111(3):631–8.

[15] Soligo M, Salvatore S, Milani R, et al. Double incontinence in urogynecologic practice: a new insight. Am J Obstet Gynecol 2003; 189(2):438–43.

[16] Nichols CM, Gill EJ, Nguyen T, et al. Anal sphincter injury in women with pelvic floor disorders. Obstet Gynecol 2004; 104(4):690–6.

[17] Chen GD, Hu SW, Chen YC, et al. Prevalence and correlations of anal incontinence and constipation in Taiwanese women. Neurourol Urodyn 2003; 22(7):664–9.

[18] Gray's Anatomy: Roger Warwick and Peter L. Williams (editors), 35th edition; Longman Group Ltd, 1973; anal musculature, 1293.

[19] Clinical Anatomy: A Revision and Applied Anatomy for Clinical Students, fifth edition, Harold Ellis (editor); Blackwell Scientific Publications, 1972; 80.

Section 2

Evaluation

Chapter 5

Practical Imaging of Faecal Incontinence: The Eyes of Science

Piloni Vittorio and Ghiselli Roberto

Additional information is available at the end of the chapter

http://dx.doi.org/10.5772/57591

1. Introduction

Faecal continence is achieved by equilibrium of several forces and a combination of factors related to stool consistency, colonic propulsion, rectal compliance and filling awareness, pelvic floor muscle reflex activity and outlet resistance. Any of these factors may be damaged and other factors can compensate for this impairment in function so that continence is ensured. Incontinence can result from the breakdown of any one or more of the mechanisms that normally ensure continence. Consequently, accurate diagnosis of all factors that interplay to cause incontinence is required in order for the condition to be treated effectively, alone or in combination, by medical or surgical management.

Until recently, diagnosis of fecal incontinence**** has relied on history taking, physical examination and anoproctoscopy. With the exception of endoanal ultrasonography (EAUS) [1-3], imaging studies have not been extensively considered as a valuable diagnostic tool for evaluating the disease, a possible explanation being that it is not easy for diagnostic imaging of the distal gut to reach the level of quality expected and achieved in most other fields of diagnosis; indeed, it demands a sufficient level of interest and commitment by the radiologist and an understanding of the inherent problems of physiology and technique. Not by chance, EAUS is traditionally performed and interpreted by the coloproctologist, who considers such an investigation the natural extension of the physical examination. Despite much controversy still in existence regarding this issue [4], recent reports have emphasized the potential role of imaging studies, including evacuation proctography, also called defecography (D) [5-7] and more recently, MR imaging of anal sphincters and the pelvic floor [8-13] in health and disease states. In particular, the development of fast-sequence MRI has renewed hope that a singular imaging study could be used to differentiate those patients requiring conservative treatment from those necessitating surgery.

The purpose of this paper is to revitalize interest for imaging studies in patients with faecal incontinence. Specifically, the paper will address aspects of technique, performance of examination and diagnostic criteria of the three modalities that are currently in use, and will select areas of their clinical application. Finally, a standard one-hour, integrated (EAUS- MR-D) imaging protocol is presented, to be applied at best in a cost-effective manner so as to have a positive impact on clinical outcomes.

2. Imaging techniques

2.1. Ultrasonography

2.1.1. Equipment

Ultrasound examination of the anal canal can be performed today by either endocavitary or external probes aided by 3D reconstruction, which provide detailed analysis of the pertinent anatomy. For the endocavitary investigation of the anal canal, called EAUS, following a digital rectal examination performed for ruling out any stenosis, a 6-16 MHz, 360° rotational transducer (type 2050, B-K medical, Herlev, Denmark) protected by a gel-containing condom and a soluble lubricant placed on the tip is gently inserted into the anus. The probe has a shaft of 270 mm, a focal length of 2-5 cm and a built-in 3D automatic motorized system allowing acquisition of up to 300 axial images over a distance of 60 mm in 60 seconds. The data from a series of 2D images are then combined to create a 3D volume displayed as a cube (Figure 1). Alternatively, the probe can be inserted into the vagina [14] to depict the anatomy of the pelvic floor and the anal canal free from distortion due to potential foreign objects (Figure 2), thus appearing similar to the image obtained during a conventional external intralabial approach. For the latter examination, a conventional 3.5-6 MHz curved array transducer is used, enabling B mode 2-D analysis or, more recently, a 3-D probe that combines an electronic curved array with mechanical sector technology, which allows fast motorized sweeps through a field of view sufficient to include the entire levator hiatus [15]. Volume data sets are then stored and displayed in the three orthogonal planes to enhance the visibility of the anatomical structure of interest.

2.1.2. Image analysis

In the axial plane, the anal sphincter complex is seen as a series of five concentric layers of different echogenicity, from inner to outer, as follows: the first hyperechoic layer corresponds to the interface of the transducer with the mucosal surface; the second layer shows an intermediate echogenicity, which results from a combination of the subepithelial tissues with the muscularis submucosa; the third hypoechoic layer corresponds to the internal anal sphincter (IAS), which is seen to extend from the anorectal junction down to 1 cm below the dentate line; the fourth layer appears as a moderately echogenic space containing a hypoechoic, thin linear structure, representing the longitudinal muscle embedded into the intersphincteric space; the fifth layer corresponds to the external anal sphincter (EAS), which shows a moderate echoge-

http://dx.doi.org/10.5772/57591

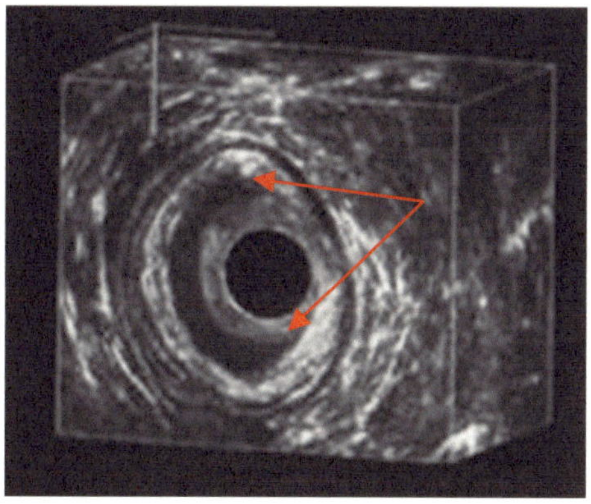

Figure 1. 3-D built-in EAUS of the anal canal with automatic image acquisition, allowing a volume of digital data to be examined: a 12-to-5 o'clock wide defect (space between the two arrows) is seen in the internal anal sphincter together with hypertrophy of the remaining portion.

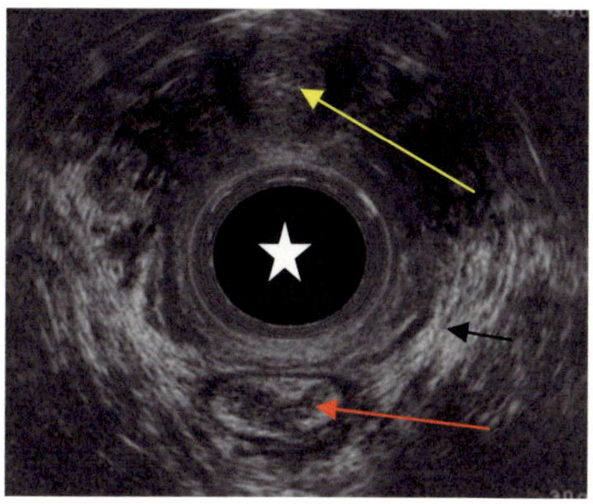

Figure 2. Endovaginal sonography performed with a 2050 B-K probe (white star) at the level of the bladder neck: the intramural portion of the urethra (yellow arrow), the anal canal (red arrow) and the pubovisceral muscle (short black arrow) are depicted.

nicity and a subdivision into a deep portion, continuous with the puborectalis muscle, a superficial portion in contact with the superficial transverse perineal muscle and a subcutaneous portion which extends below the IAS. Via the transvaginal or the transperineal route, the undisturbed virtual lumen of the anal canal is also seen at the centre as a "X-shaped" hypoechoic structure representing the mucosa (Figure 3a and b). Each couple of contiguous branches in this X image delimits three to four triangular hyperechoic structures representing the submucosa. On the longitudinal planes, the anal canal shows a railroad-like appearance of different echogenic structures, which exactly reproduces that described in the axial planes. The normal IAS is between 2 to 3 mm thick and the normal EAS in between 4 to 5 mm thick. The IAS becomes thicker and more hyperechoic with age, probably reflecting collagen replacement. Conversely, the EAS tends to become thinner with age. For female patients being evaluated for faecal incontinence, the examination is occasionally performed with the patient in the prone position to more clearly delineate the anterior aspect of the EAS and improve visualization of the perineum.

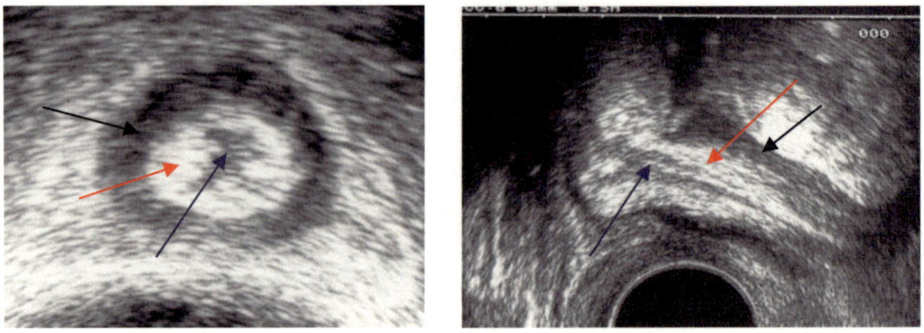

(a) (b)

Figure 3. Two-dimensional (2-D) translabial imaging of the anal canal obtained with a 3.5 MHz convex probe showing the continuous hypoechoic ring of internal anal sphincter (black arrow), the hyperechoic submucosa (red arrow) and the "X-shaped" hypoechoic mucosa (blue arrow) in the axial view (a) and in the sagittal view (b)

2.1.2.1. Diagnostic criteria

The role of EAUS in faecal incontinence is specifically related to the detection of anal sphincter lesions including tear, scarring, thinning and atrophy. More particularly, the term 'tear' is used to indicate any discontinuity in the sphincter layer, which is seen as a break of the normal echotexture and geometrical configuration. On the other hand, the term 'scarring' relates to the presence of focal changes in echogenicity, which alter the expected normal pattern. 'Thinning' and "atrophy are virtually synonymous at sonography, which has no other criteria than a reduction in the thickness of the muscle bulk to make the diagnosis. At EAUS, defects in the IAS appear as hyperechoic breaks [16] in the normally hypoechoic ring, as opposed to defects in the EAS, which appear as relatively hypoechoic areas in the normally hyperechoic ring (Figure 4a and b). According to Starck [17, 18], a discontinuity involving less than half the thickness of the EAS and/or the IAS **should not** be classified as a defect. The term "partial defect" is used to indicate discontinuities engaging at least half sphincter thickness, while "total defect" is assigned when the whole sphincter thickness is involved. In order to define the severity of the lesion, sphincter defects are measured and classified taking into account their location as well as the longitudinal and circumferential extension. Traditionally, the site of the defect is described by referring to the "anal clock", which is the view of the anal sphincter complex with the patient in the lithotomy position, where 12 o'clock is the anterior perineum, six o'clock is the natal cleft, three o'clock is the left lateral aspect and nine o'clock is the right of the anal canal. The starting point of the defect and quantification of how many hours (or degrees) it extends clockwise are registered together with annotation of its longitudinal extension, i.e., whether involving half the sphincter length, more than half, or the whole length.

http://dx.doi.org/10.5772/57591

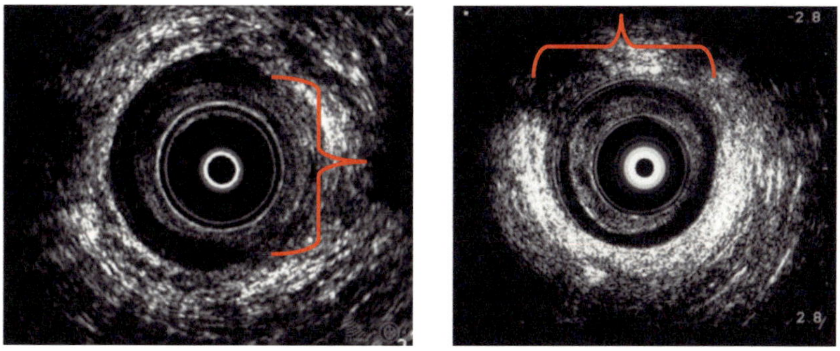

(a) (b)

Figure 4. Close-up view of the anal sphincters at EAUS in the axial plane from two different patients: typical sonographic feature of the internal (a) and the external (b) anal sphincter defect which are seen as wide gaps (parenthesis) filled by fibrotic tissue showing moderate echogenicity and inhomogeneous hypoechogenicity, respectively. (Courtesy of dr. Favetta U.)

2.1.2.2. Diagnostic accuracy

Thanks to its superior axial resolution of less than 0.1 mm and lateral resolution of 0.8 mm in the focus zone, together with a slice thickness for reconstruction of 0.2 mm allowing a voxel size of 0.2 mm^3, 3-D EAUS gives the most accurate assessment of anal sphincter anatomy and may significantly improve the diagnostic confidence of detecting damage to the anal sphincter complex [19]. The examination, performed immediately after vaginal delivery, allows diagnosis of clinically undetected anal sphincter tears that might be associated with subsequent faecal incontinence with a reported positive predict value of 37% [20]. When compared to other modern imaging techniques, the diagnostic accuracy between EAUS and endoanal MRI performed on the same day has been evaluated in 52 patients with faecal incontinence in comparison with clinical examination and anorectal physiological testing [21]. Complete agreement between the two techniques was found in 32 and disagreement in 20, with incorrect interpretation (arbitration) in six on anal ultrasound and in 15 on endoanal MR, and only one error made on sonography vs. 12 errors on MR when evaluating the IAS, as opposed to five errors vs. six, respectively, when evaluating the EAS. The authors concluded that anal endoanal sonography is a better imaging modality for evaluating IAS injury, while sonography and MRI have equivalent results in the evaluation of EAS injury.

3. Defecography

Despite the recent advent of high-technology modalities and the drawback of somatic and genetic risks associated with radiation exposure, conventional (X-ray) defecography (D) still has enduring value as a diagnostic test in FI. Contrary to the general view that the examination is difficult to perform in these patients, because they are unable to hold the injected rectal contrast, D can be performed in virtually any patient who can have his/her ampulla filled with barium paste, be placed on a sitting chair and instructed to pass and stop the barium stream on command. The procedure is not time-consuming, requires intermittent and infrequent fluoroscopy or film taking and its diagnostic yield maintains a prominent role with great clinical and therapeutic implications. Several aspects of the technique, which has been described previously [6], help to obtain a uniformly satisfactory outcome of the examination as follows:

Imaging Technique: examinations are carried out on an all-purpose gastrointestinal tract remote controlled X-ray unit (Opera T90e model, General Medical Merate, Bergamo, Italy), using the video outlet from the monitor to record the fluoroscopic images onto a digital imaging system. Technical parameters include the following: voltage, 120 kV; mA, 2; field of view, 170 cm^2 (continuous fluoroscopy) and voltage, 75kV; mA, 400; number of images, 1Fps; number of series, 5 (digital radiography). For the examination, a radiopaque ruler is attached to the table to enable subsequent calculation of distances and angles from the images. A suspension of 400 grams of powder containing barium sulphate (Pronto Bario Colon, Bracco Laboratories, Milan, Italy) is gradually diluted in 160 mL of water heated at body temperature, resulting in a mixture that has the consistency of semisolid faeces. With the patient lying in the left lateral decubitus position on the radiological table and a pad positioned under the exposed buttocks to collect any material, the unprepared rectum is filled with up to 180 mL of this mixture, unless anticipated leakage occurs. The barium paste is introduced slowly through the anal canal via a 3 mm wide catheter connected to a 60 mL syringe. In case of barium loss, the injection is discontinued and the first image series is started immediately with the patient still lying on his/her left side; the first leakage volume and the total amount of contrast retained are registered; fluoroscopy is also continued while tilting the table upright (Figure 5a and b) during the patient's attempt to interrupt the barium stream (stop test). At this point, the patient is seated on a water-filled commode placed on the table's footrest after having adjusted a single use, removable plastic bag located directly within the commode. Four standard series of images are then taken at rest, squeeze, strain and emptying in sequential order. Permanent records and measurements of established parameters are obtained, including the anorectal angle (ARA°), the rectal and anal maximum diameters and the position of the anorectal junction (ARJ), with respect to the lower margin of the ischial tuberosities taken as reference. At the end of the examination, the review of defecographic series is performed by the examiner from the same console for assessment and reporting.

Image Analysis: the following observations are made from defecograms:

- Rectal size, i.e., measurement of maximum anteroposterior diameter from lateral view at capacity as an index of rectal compliance.

- Anal width, i.e., maximal distance between the two inner margins of the anal canal measured at rest in the total absence of efforts to void as an index of the closing mechanism of the anal sphincter.

http://dx.doi.org/10.5772/57591

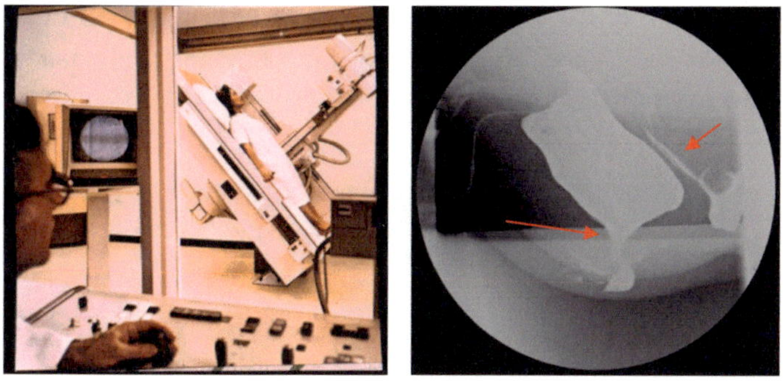

(a) (b)

Figure 5. Continuous fluoroscopic monitoring at defecography while tilting the patient upright (a) for evidence of incontinence: a wider than normal 115° resting anorectal angle (long arrow) is seen (b) together with barium leak and failure of anal wall apposition. The short arrow points at the contrast within the vaginal canal injected as anatomical landmark.

- ARA°, defined as the angle between the longitudinal axis of the anal canal and a line drawn tangent to the posterior margin of the rectal ampulla close to the ARJ as an index of the activity of the puborectalis muscle.

- The position of the pelvic floor, defined as the perpendicular distance of the ARJ from the lower margin of the ischial tuberosities; ARJ upward/downward mobility during squeezing, coughing and straining, respectively, is taken as an index of tonic and reflex activity of the levator ani muscle as a whole.

- Barium loss, defined as any incompetence to the average 180 mL amount of the injected rectal contrast. The first leakage volume and the total amount injected before leakage are registered.

- The presence of associated pathologies, including mucosal prolapse, rectocele, rectoanal intussusception and excessive descent of the ARJ are also registered.

Diagnostic Criteria: most common findings associated with faecal incontinence include (a) **inability to retain the contrast material**, also called *barium loss* signs, with or without awareness of it. This is graded as minor (+) when it occurs only with the patient seated during coughing and/or straining forcefully, moderate (++) when it occurs during tilting the table upright or sitting at rest and straining minimally, and severe (+++) when it occurs with the patient still lying during retrograde injection; (b) **lack of apposition of anal walls** at rest, also called *anal gaping*, leading the contrast medium to fill the anal canal, which shows a mean transverse diameter ≥ 10 mm as a sign of incompetence; (c) **abnormal rectal size**, i.e., > 7.5 cm in case of rectal inertia and faecaloma or < 4 cm in case of overactive hyper-reflective ampulla; (d) **poor squeezing and stop test**, seen as inability or fatiguing when asked to actively contract the pelvic floor musculature and anal sphincter ; (e) **obtuse ARA°** at rest > 116°; (f) **associated abnormalities** such as (1) descent of the ARJ > 4 cm below the ischial tuberosities; (2) full-thickness rectoanal intussusception (Figure 6a and b), defined as an intraluminal filling defect

> 1 cm in diameter, showing distal progression on evacuation; (3) rectocele, defined as any bulging of the anterior rectal wall greater than 2 cm beyond the expected line extending upward through the anterior margin of the anal canal.

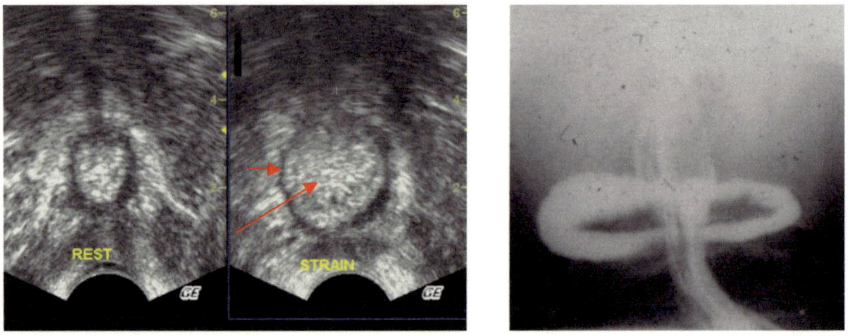

(a) (b)

Figure 6. Sixty-two year-old woman under pharmacological treatment for psychological depression, with history of obstetric trauma, chronic constipation and episodes of passive fecal incontinence of recent onset. Integrated diagnostic work-up including perineal sonography (a) and defecography (b) within the same session: at sonography, thinning of the internal anal sphincter (short arrow) on straining and significant increase of the submucosal space (long arrow) suggestive of full-thickness intussusception. At defecography, involuntary barium loss during retrograde injection (not shown) and evidence of rectoanal intussusception with typical "Saturn's ring" sign due to entrapment of contrast on emptying within the double layer mucosa infolding.

Diagnostic Accuracy: the " barium loss" sign occurring at rest has been found [22] to be at the receiver operating curve (ROC) analysis a highly reliable index of faecal incontinence (specificity 93-100%, intraobserver agreement *K* value 0.82, *Z* 21.58, $p < 0.001$) with a false-negative rate of 14.2% limited to patients with minor episodes of incontinence only. Useful adjunctive criteria include an anal diameter > 10 mm at rest and a poor stop test. Additionally, irrespective of age, gender and associated abnormalities, namely rectal prolapse, the resting ARA° measurement could reliably be reinterpreted and allowed for good differentiation between continent and incontinent subjects [23]. More precisely, it was found to be the most discriminating index at ANOVA by Fisher's test (104.5°± 10.3 vs 116.2° ± 23.6, *F* 9.4, $p < 0.01$), with an accuracy of 79%, false-positive rate of 15.3% and false-negative rate of 26.5%. Abnormal rectal size and filling sensation (altered compliance) and rectoanal intussusception (obstructed defecation syndrome) helped the clinician in the search for an aetiologic diagnosis.

4. Magnetic resonance

Several studies have used static and dynamic high-resolution MR imaging to assess pelvic organ prolapse and anal sphincter derangements [24-30]. Without the hazard of ionizing radiation, this technique provides excellent depiction of the anal sphincter complex and all perianal spaces, including a multiplanar global evaluation of fat recesses, ligaments, fascial attachments and the pelvic floor musculature. As such, MR imaging is preferable in young persons who are in their reproductive age. In addition, the development of fast sequence imaging since the early 90s has allowed for also including the assessment of voiding and evacuation phenomenon, leading to the so called MR-defecography as an alternative to the conventional (X-ray) examination. A potential disadvantage of MR, when compared to D, is its less physiologic nature, because the examination is usually performed with the patient supine. On the other hand, it provides superior reproducibility when measuring the parameters of anorectal configuration [31, 32].

Imaging Technique: in our centre, MR imaging is routinely performed in subjects with faecal incontinence with a conventional 1.5 T horizontally-oriented magnet system (Philips, Achieva model, The Netherlands), using an external body SENSE and a four-channel phased array coil wrapped around the patient's pelvis. In order to depict the morphology and quantify the thickness of the sphincter complex free from distortion, a flexible rubber catheter 3 mm in diameter is inserted at the beginning through the anus to act as a luminal marker and for subsequent contrast administration (acoustic gel). Static T2-weighted images of the pelvic region are acquired first in the sagittal plane using fast spin echo (FSE) pulse sequence (TR/TE, 3704/90 ms; FOV, 32 cm; slice thickness, 4 mm; interslice gap, 0.6 mm; ETL, 18; matrix size, 444x310 ; BW, 125.24 kHz; NEX, 4; FA°, 90) so as to define the field of view and put into focus the intra-anal marker. Subsequent axial and coronal images of the anal sphincter complex and pertinent perianal anatomy are acquired with the same pulse sequence and sections obtained parallel and transverse to the long axis of the anal canal. Thereafter, without interruption during scanning or patient movement, up to 160 mL of acoustic gel is slowly injected via the catheter by the examiner unless early leakage of contrast occurs. After probe withdrawal and proper patient coaching, dynamic images are obtained at rest, on squeezing, maximal straining and emptying in the midsagittal plane using a T1-weighted, balance fast field echo (BFFE) pulse sequence (TR/TE, 2.8/1.39 ms; FOV 300x300; section thickness, 30 mm; BW, 125.0 kHz; matrix size, 160x 160; acquisition time, one image/0.891sec over 48 sec; NEX, 2). The same sequence is then repeated during evacuation in the coronal plane centred over the anorectal junction. Finally, three parallel, contiguous 1-cm-thick sections, using the same pulse sequence (TR/TE, 3/1.51 ms; NEX, two acquisition time, nine sec) are obtained in the axial plane starting at the upper margin of the pubic symphysis down to the level of the anal margin to image the levator hiatus during the Valsalva manoeuvre in a steady state.

Image Analysis: key images for interpretation of the anal sphincter complex anatomy are those obtained in the midcoronal plane (Figure 7), which allows for good distinction between the innermost muscle layer of the internal anal sphincter showing intermediate signal intensity and the outer low signal intensity layer of the external sphincter. The latter also shows a characteristic shape, i.e., at its lower end it is seen to fold inward and upward to form a double layer leaving space to the terminal fibres of the longitudinal muscle, while at its upper and outer margin a cleft is clearly visible, which separates it from the puborectalis muscle. Coronal sections obtained slightly anterior and posterior to the midplane offer good depiction of the urogenital diaphragm, superficial and deep perineal muscles, ischiocavernosus muscle and levator ani muscle, respectively. In the axial plane, the internal sphincter is a ring-like hyperintense structure surrounded by the hypointense external sphincter with the interposition of the relatively hyperintense intersphincteric space; key images for interpretation are those taken at the midportion of the anal canal where the two halves of the external anal sphincters become connected to each other. In the midsagittal plane, the anococcygeal ligament connects the external sphincter to the coccygeal bone and separates the superficial from the deep post-anal plane. Anteriorly, the puborectalis muscle and the bulbocavernous muscle are seen to support the external sphincter. Overall, the anal canal shows a cylindrical appearance, averaging 5.7cm in length with a mean thickness of 2.3 mm for the internal sphincter, 1.3 mm for the longitudinal muscle and 3.4 mm for the external sphincter. The anal sphincter's MR *signal intensity* is also given great relevance and compared to that of the obturator internus muscle, being described as the same (normal), higher (fibro-fatty degeneration) or lower (scarring). MR image analysis of the whole pelvis also includes (a) measurement of the width of the levator hiatus in the axial plane on straining at the point of its maximum extension at the level of the bladder neck and proximal urethra. For this, a contour tracking technique, allowing for anatomically adapted and automatically placed region of interest (ROI) is employed. A hiatal area of less than 25 cm^2 on Valsalva is reported to be consistent with normal pelvic support; (b) evaluation of pelvic organs' mobility in the midsagittal plane on Valsalva, by calculating the vertical distance of the bladder base, the cervix or vaginal cuff and the rectal floor from the pubococcygeal line (PCL) drawn from the lower border of the symphisis pubis to the last joint of the coccyx. According to Fielding, [28] pelvic organ descent beyond this line should not exceed 1 cm; (c) measurement of the levator plate angle (LPA) relative to a horizontal reference line; average values of 44.3° are reported [29] in women with normal support.

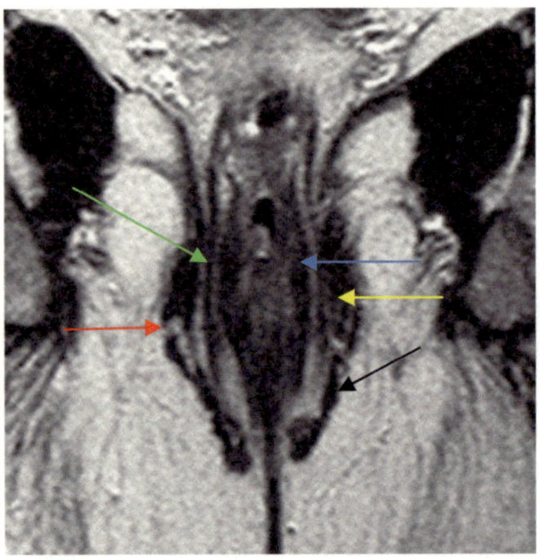

Figure 7. Forty-eight-year-old man with prior fistulotomy (red arrow) and no evidence of fecal incontinence. Postoperative mid coronal T 2-weighted MRI with external coil showing preserved integrity of the sphincter complex including the internal sphincter (sky-blue arrow), the external sphincter (black arrow), and the longitudinal muscle (green arrow). Incidentally, focal areas of increased signal intensity are observed within the puborectalis muscle (yellow arrow) consistent with fibrofatty degeneration.

Diagnostic Criteria: the MR diagnosis of anal sphincter derangement in faecal incontinence is two-fold and relies on: 1) a < 2 mm thinning of the internal anal sphincter for age > 50 years, which is considered consistent with **degeneration** of the muscle and responsible for passive

http://dx.doi.org/10.5772/57591

faecal incontinence; 2) disruption of the sphincteric ring with or without loss of striated muscle bulk and fat replacement, which are typical findings of external sphincter **tears and atrophy** most often associated with childbirth trauma, incisional surgery and dilatation procedures. Occasionally, degeneration and atrophy concur to maintain faecal incontinence even after surgical implant of bulking agents (Figure 8a and b). In symptomatic patients, pelvic organs descent greater than 2 cm below the PCL (Figure 9) is considered an indication of **pelvic floor laxity**, requiring surgical intervention. More precisely, quantification of **pelvic organ prolapse** by MR imaging has been classified [25] as mild if the vertical distance from the PCL on maximum straining extends for less than 3 cm (grades 1-2 of the Baden-Walker classification), moderate if it is between 3 and 6 cm (Baden-Walker grade 3) and severe if it exceeds 6 cm (Baden-Walker grade 3-4). Further characterization of the dysfunction and evidence of pelvic organ impingement (Figure 10) can be derived from a levator **hiatus area** of 30-34.9 cm^2 (mild), 35-39.9 cm^2 (moderate) and ≥40 cm^2 (marked ballooning), respectively [15]. Furthermore, with respect to controls, women with prolapse have been reported [11] to exhibit a significant + 21% **more vertical levator plate** with average LPA° of 53.4° vs 44.3°. Most common associated abnormalities seen during the expulsion of rectal contrast include **rectocele**, which is classified as mild when its protrusion from the expected anterior rectal wall is less than 2 cm, moderate if 2-4 cm and severe if greater than 4 cm, as well as **intussusception**, which is termed intrarectal (grade 1) when it remains within the rectum, intra-anal (grade 2) if its apex penetrates the proximal half of the anal canal, intra-anal (grade 3), if the apex is seen to impinge on the distal half of the anal canal and external (grade 4) if it is extruded outward.

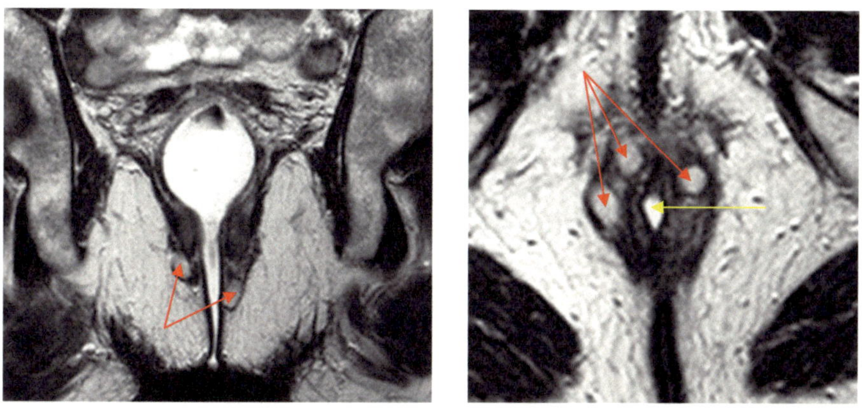

(a) (b)

Figure 8. MR- defecographic images obtained in the coronal (a) and axial(b) plane in a sixty-one-year-old woman with persistent fecal incontinence after multiple gate keeper implants (red arrows) for degeneration of the internal sphincter and atrophy/disruption of the external sphinter: involuntary loss of contrast and lack of anal wall apposition (yellow arrow).

Diagnostic Accuracy: despite their limited availability, endoanal MR coils have been used as an alternative to EAUS with comparable results for detection of anal sphincter defects and a clear superiority of MRI for EAS atrophy [33, 34]. However, high-resolution MRI using external

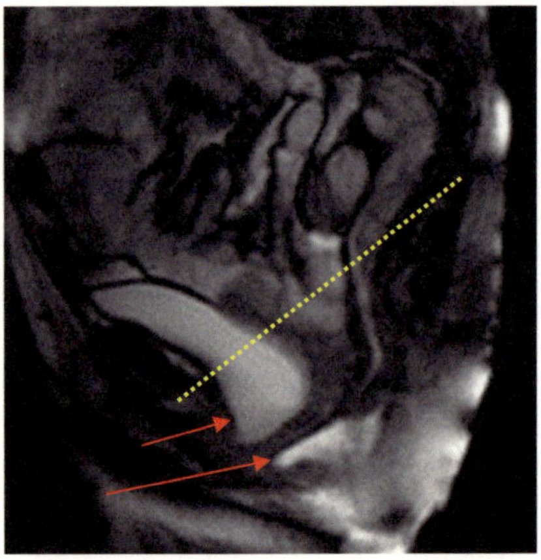

Figure 9. Mid- sagittal MR-defecographic series with BFFE T 1-weighted pulse sequence: excessive descent of the bladder base (short red arrow) and rectal floor (long red arrow) on straining below the pubococcygeal line (yellow dotted line) due to pelvic floor laxity in a thirty-one year-old woman with chronic strain at stool and staining episodes.

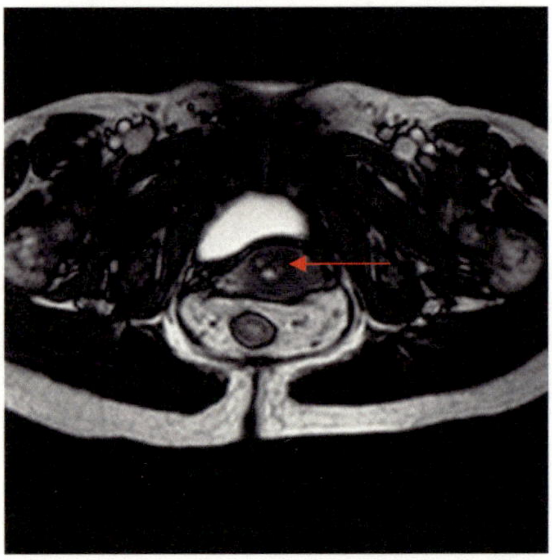

Figure 10. Dynamic MR- defecography in the axial plane at the level of the lower margin of the symphysis pubis: ballooning of the levator hiatus with impingement of the uterine cervix (red arrow) between the prolapsed bladder base, anteriorly and the anorectum, posteriorly.

phased-array coils in patients with faecal incontinence has the advantage of simultaneously providing both structural and functional information on the pelvic floor structures and anal sphincter complex. In our experience, the potential advantage of this technique is highlighted by its ability to be as accurate as EAUS in detecting structural changes of the sphincteric such as tears, atrophy and areas of focal degeneration and disruption, together with offering contemporary evidence of functional derangements including an inefficient anal closing mechanism with involuntary loss of rectal contrast and pelvic floor laxity. Until now, however there has been no mention of comparative studies of external coil MRI with EAUS and endoanal MRI in faecal incontinence published in the literature.

http://dx.doi.org/10.5772/57591

5. Clinical application of diagnostic imaging in faecal incontinence

From a practical point of view, one may consider the application of imaging studies to be worth pursuing in at least three situations as follows:

a. Following surgical pelvic floor reconstruction in the neonatal period for congenital anomalies such as anal atresia, imperforate anus, bicornuate uterus, persistent vaginal septum and associated urologic or sacrococcygeal anomalies, male and female subjects are at increased risk for developing faecal incontinence in adult life [35], particularly on physical exertion, heavy work activity or in case of pregnancy. Usually, because such patients are infants when operated on, it often takes many years before full evaluation of results for a given anomaly can be given. Today, when considering long-term results of surgery with regard to anorectal adequacy and continence, we are looking for more than operative survival or a complication-free postoperative course. In an attempt to assess the patient's function or adjustment to his/her disability, a complete imaging investigation [36] is highly recommended, including EAUS and pelvic MRI: these two noninvasive diagnostic tools permit clear depiction of postoperative pelvic floor anatomy and detection of even subtle sphincter derangements that might interfere with future activities.

b. Damage to the anal sphincter from vaginal delivery is a common cause of faecal incontinence in middle-aged women. The muscle tears, which may involve one or both parts of the sphincter, are situated consistently in the anterior quadrant. After vaginal delivery, women have typically been reported to undergo anal sphincter tears in between 0.36% and 8.4% of cases [17], even though small anal sphincter defects and minor gas incontinence are also occasionally found in nulliparous women without known sphincter trauma. However, only one third of these women will develop faecal incontinence and only of a minor degree, despite being treated with primary sphincter repair soon after delivery. Flatus incontinence after vaginal delivery is also described to be more common in women with sphincter disruption compared to those who received an episiotomy or a caesarean section (58.6%, 30.3% and 15.2%, respectively). While the use of EAUS from one day to six months after childbirth is mainly focused on the detection of sphincter disruption, MR imaging is better suited to quantify systematic changes occurring in the levator ani muscle (LA), including focal areas of increased signal intensity (i.e., fibrofatty degeneration), reduced thickness, LA muscle avulsion and tears, detachment from the endopelvic fascia and perineal body disruption and descent. All of these are considered to be highly correlated with the development of pelvic organ prolapse (POP) and double incontinence after the fifth decade.

c. Patients who are about to undergo *elective anorectal surgery* with major procedures such as total colectomy and ileo-anal anastomosis (ulcerative colitis, familial polyposis), low coloanal anastomosis (rectal tumour), or more common procedures such as haemorrhoidectomy, fistulectomy, rectopexy and rectocele repair (prolapsed haemorrhoids, anal-perianal sepsis, intussusceptions and rectal prolapse) are potential candidates for developing faecal urgency and becoming more or less incontinent to faeces after surgery. This can occur for two reasons: mainly a reduced rectal reservoir function and/or anal sphincter injury. In particular it should be noted that the internal sphincter muscle fibres, which contribute about 80% of the resting anal tone, are usually adhered to and easily dragged up with haemorrhoidal tissues during haemorrhoidectomy, leading to frequent episodes of post-operative mucous discharge and passive incontinence unless a substantial amount of vascular cushions and bridges of anoderm are preserved [37]. With regard to perianal sepsis, the overall incidence of major faecal incontinence after surgical management of complex fistulas is estimated at approximately 7%. While no effect is generally noted on continence in patients treated for low fistulae, minor incontinence can occur in up to 33% in patients in whom the sphincter muscle is divided after two-stage fistulotomy or cutting using the seton technique. Regardless of the pathology and the procedure being used, the patient's sphincter adequacy should be carefully assessed before and after surgery. A combination of EAUS, D and pelvic MRI study is needed to rule out a number of abnormalities such as anal sphincter defects, dehiscences, sinus tracts and abscesses, granulomas, strictures of the anastomotic ring, small uncompliant (neo) rectum and anal gaping.

6. Algorithm and integrated diagnostic work-up

EAUS is the most important imaging test to start with and to provide information about the morphology of a potentially disrupted sphincter. As a second step, in order to select patients for sphincteroplasty, an MRI with an external coil will help to identify focal areas of atrophy and fat replacement of the anal sphincter complex, which US tests does not identify. MR defecography is also an unsurpassed modality for depicting associated abnormalities such as pelvic organ prolapse, intra-anal intussusception, rectocele, pelvic floor weakness and pudendal nerve neuropathy. Finally, D is occasionally useful for sorting out overflow faecal incontinence and/or hyperactive, uncompliant rectal ampulla. For better patient compliance and quicker diagnostic algorithm, in the presence of adequate expertise and instruments, it is technically possible to perform a complete and integrated imaging investigation, i.e., EAUS + MR ± D, within the same session in less than one-hour, as follows:

1. 2D or 3D EAUS is performed first for proper detection and staging of any anal sphincter damage. For the examination, the patient lies on his/her left side. The lubricated probe is gently inserted into the rectal ampulla for acquisition of the images from the volume of interest. Average time to complete the examination is between 10 and 15 minutes, which includes patient preparation and positioning, image acquisition, interpretation and reporting.

2. The patient is then moved into the MR imaging diagnostic room to undergo both static and dynamic pelvic floor examination with external coil. Usually, after coaching the patient and full explanation of the finality of the examination, a standard dose of contrast (acoustic gel) is administered. Average time for the examination, image interpretation and measurements of recognized parameters is between 25 and 30 minutes.

3. If necessary, the patient is then positioned horizontally on the X-ray table of a remote controlled diagnostic unit to undergo D, which includes (a) radiopaque contrast administration and tilting upright after probe withdrawal under continuous fluoroscopic control; (b) positioning seated on a specially designed commode; (c) image acquisition and recording in the lateral and anteroposterior plane. The required average time is 10 minutes.

7. Reporting

All reports on imaging techniques should specify the position of the patient during image acquisition as well as the performance of specific manoeuvres according to the examiner's demand. When using ultrasonography, detailed information is given concerning the transducer type, orientation and route of scanning; for magnetic resonance imaging, specifics of the technique include the equipment used, plane of imaging, pulse sequences, scan time, use and type of contrast, measurements and parameters during image analysis. Static and dynamic contrast radiography should include a description of the type, timing and amount of contrast administration and sequence of organ opacification, projections and exposures. Finally, a short and concise list of the abnormalities observed is included, followed by the most likely hypothesis of the (possible) mechanism responsible for the disease and suggestions regarding further investigation.

8. Combined non-imaging studies

Traditionally, anorectal manometry [38], i.e., calculation of the longitudinal pressure profile of the anal canal and, more recently, anal vector volume analysis [39] have received great consideration in the diagnostic work-up of faecal incontinence, being simple and relatively cheap procedures that help to indicate the exact location of any focal reduction in pressure along the course of a disrupted anal sphincter. More particularly, the validity of anal pressure vectography [40] should be emphasized in combination with EAUS or endoanal magnetic resonance [41], since it allows for evaluation of the radial pressure in the anal canal from which a symmetry index can be obtained that more closely reflects the functional relevance of any proven defect in anatomical integrity. However, factors other than anal sphincter muscles contributing to the pressure generated within the anal canal, such as the puborectalis muscle, should also be considered as a possible cause of incorrect vectorgram. Besides providing data on the responsibility of the internal and external anal sphincter in causing faecal incontinence, anorectal manometry is useful for demonstrating a reduced capacity and compliance of the rectum, as well as a reduced sensation and reflex activity of the anorectum, by correlating findings of the pressure profile with those from defecographic series. On assessing patients with possible neurogenic aetiology of their incontinence, electrodiagnostic tests should be considered [42], including electromyography (EMG) and a pudendal nerve terminal motor latency (PNTML) test. By EMG, the electrical activity arising in the external anal sphincter and puborectalis muscle at rest, straining and during voluntary contraction is recorded and measurements are performed of the amplitude, duration and number of phases of motor unit action potentials, with inference on the innervations and functional state within the muscle. PNTML, on the other hand, evaluates conduction time in the motor nerve fibres of the pelvic floor musculature by recording the time interval from nerve stimulation to the onset of the electrical response in the muscle. Most common changes in EMG activity include denervation, which leads to loss of responsiveness and atrophy of the affected fibres and reinnervation occurring either by regrowth of the damaged axons or by sprouting of nearby unaffected axons, with a tendency for fibres to be clustered together in small groups; this change in spatial distribution will lead to a variation in the amplitude and duration of motor unit action potentials recorded by EMG. While denervated muscle fibres may show spontaneous activity at rest, evidence of reinnervation is offered by an increase in motor unit potential parameters. At PNTML, a prolonged latency has been reported in faecal incontinence, obstetric trauma and perineal descent; this parameter was also proposed as a predictive factor for the clinical outcome of biofeedback therapy or surgical repair, despite it being less sensitive for showing anal sphincter denervation when compared to needle EMG and a lack of correlation with manometric pressure studies. Finally, somatosensory evoked potentials (SEPs) and mucosal sensitivity (MS) to thermal or electrical stimulation of the anal canal have been proposed to reveal a lesion affecting the large-diameter nerve fibres in patients with suspected sensory deficit in the perineum and measuring anal sensation, respectively. Magnetic resonance imaging of pudendal nerve [43] is the only diagnostic tool that has been described as potentially useful in patients with positive electrodiagnostic test results.

9. Conclusions

Until some decades ago, the major examination method for patients with faecal incontinence has relied on history taking, physical inspection and digital examination. Most commonly, questioning about the nature of incontinence (passive vs. urgency) is the initial diagnostic step that helps to further delineate various causes. Passive incontinence usually indicates a defect in sphincter muscle integrity, loss of sphincter innervation with pelvic floor laxity, or decreased rectal sensation. On the other hand, urgency followed by incontinence is most frequently associated with a problem concerning rectal compliance due to colitis, prior surgery or radiation. Today, Diagnostic imaging is more and more frequently considered in subsequent evaluation, with important therapeutic implications.. A firm understanding of factors contributing to the image is helpful in the performance of the examination, but is also essential for accurate interpretation. EAUS is mandatory for detection of anal sphincter defects. Thereafter, static and dynamic pelvic MRI with external coil is an integral part of the investigation for assessment of associated pelvic floor disorders and better characterization of sphincter atrophy. D is occasionally useful to offer objective documentation of the inability to retain rectal content. Although many aspects of faecal incontinence remain obscure, imaging studies may contribute to patient management and clinical decision-making.

http://dx.doi.org/10.5772/57591

Acknowledgements

The authors are especially indebted to Mrs A. Donzelli, English language teacher, for her assistance in reviewing the manuscript and to Dr U. Favetta, surgeon, for providing some of the illustrations.

Author details

Piloni Vittorio[1] and Ghiselli Roberto[2]

*Address all correspondence to: vittorio.piloni@libero.it

1 Pelvic Floor Imaging Centre. Villa Silvia Clinic, Senigallia (AN), Italy

2 Department of Surgery University of Ancona, United Hospitals "Umberto I , GM. Lancisi, G. Salesi", Ancona, Italy

References

[1] Frudinger A, Bartram CI, Halligan S et al. Examination techniques for endosonography of the anal canal. Abdom Imaging 1998; 23:301-303.

[2] Gold DM, Bartram C, Halligan S et al. Three-dimensional endoanal sonography in assessing anal canal injury. Br J Surg 1999; 86:365-370.

[3] Bartram CI. Functional anorectal imaging. Abdominal Imaging 2005; 30:195-203.

[4] Baeten C, Bartolo DCC, Lehur PA et al. Consensus conference on faecal incontinence. Tech Coloproctol 2007; 11:225-233.

[5] Piloni V, Ascoli G, Marmorale C. Contribution of defecography to the diagnosis of faecal incontinence. Coloproctology 1988; 10:297-301.

[6] Piloni V. Defecography. Transit times and imaging techniques. In Romano G. (ed). Diagnosis and treatment of fecal incontinence. Idelson-Gnocchi pub, ISBN 10:192864919X; 2000; 6: 81-98.

[7] Stoker J, Bartram CI, Halligan S. Imaging of the posterior pelvic floor. Eur Radiol 2002; 12:779-788.

[8] Hussain SM, Stoker J, Lameris JS. Anal sphincter complex: endoanal MR imaging of normal anatomy. Radiology 1995; 197:671-677.

[9] Healy JC, Halligan S, Reznek RH et al. Patterns of prolapse in women with symptoms of pelvic floor weakness: assessment with MR imaging. Radiology 1997; 203:77-81.

[10] Beets-Tan RG, Beets GL, van der Hoop AG et al. High-resolution magnetic resonance imaging of the anorectal region without an endocoil. Abdom Imaging 1999; 24:576-581.

[11] Tunn R, DeLancey JOL, Howard D et al. MR imaging of levator ani muscle recovery following vaginal delivery. Int Urogynecol J 1999; 10:300-307.

[12] Tunn R, DeLancey JOL, Quint EE. Visibility of pelvic organ support system structures in magnetic resonance images without an endovaginal coil. Am J Obstet Gynecol 2001; 184:1156-1163.

[13] Williams AB, Molouf AD, Bartram CI et al. Assessment of external anal sphincter morphology in idiopathic fecal incontinence with endocoil magnetic resonance imaging. Dig Dis Sci, 2001; 46:1466-1471.

[14] Santoro GA, Di Falco G. Three-dimensional endoluminal ultrasonography. In Santoro GA, Wieczorek AP, Bartram CI (eds). Pelvic floor disorders. Springer-Verlag Italia, 2010; 24:285-296.

[15] Dietz HP, Shek C, Clarcke B. Biometry of the pubovisceral muscle and levator hiatus by three-dimensional pelvic floor ultrasound. Ultrasound Obstet Gynecol 2005; 25:580-585.

[16] Santoro GA, Di Falco G. Endoanal and endorectal ultrasonography: methodology and normal pelvic floor anatomy. In Santoro GA, Wieczorek AP, Bartram CI (eds). Pelvic floor disorders Springer-Verlag Italia, 2010; 8:91-102.

[17] Starck M, Bohe M, Valentin L. Results of endosonographic imaging of the anal sphincter 2-7 days after primary repair of third-or-fourth-degree obstetric sphincter tears. Ultrasound Obstet Gynecol 2003; 22:609-615.

[18] Starck M, Bohe M, Fortling B et al. Endosonography of the anal sphincter in women of different ages and parity. Ultrasound Obstet Gynecol 2005; 25:169-176.

[19] Christensen AF, Nyhuus B, Nielsen MB et al. Three-dimensional anal endosonography may improve diagnostic confidence of detecting damage to the anal sphincter complex. Br J Radiol 2005; 78:308-311.

[20] Faltin DL, Boulvain M, Irion O et al. Diagnosis of anal sphincter tears by postpartum endosonography to predict fecal incontinence. Obstet Gynecol 2000; 95:643-647

[21] Malouf AJ, Williams AB, Halligan S et al. Prospective assessment of accuracy of endoanal MR imaging and endosonography in patients with fecal incontinence. Am J Roentgenol 2000; 175:741-745.

[22] Piloni V, Gesuita R, Fioravanti P et al. Diagnosis of fecal incontinence by defecography: receiver operating characteristic (ROC) analysis. Tech Coloproct 1995; 2:70-72.

[23] Piloni V, Fioravanti P, Spazzafumo L et al. Measurement of the anorectal angle by defecography for the diagnosis of fecal incontinence. Int J Colorect Dis 1999; 14:131-135.

[24] DeLancey JOL, Hurd WW. Size of the urogenital hiatus in the levator ani muscles in normal women and women with pelvic organ prolapse. Obstet Gynecol 1988; 91:364-368.

[25] Comiter CV, Vasavada SP, Barbaric ZL et al. Grading pelvic prolapse and pelvic floor relaxation using dynamic magnetic resonance imaging. Urology 1999; 54(3): 454-457.

[26] Kelvin FM, Maglinte DDT, Hale DS et al. Female pelvic organ prolapse: a comparison of triphasic dynamic MR imaging and triphasic fluoroscopic cystocolpoproctography. Am J Roentgenol 2000; 174: 81-88.

[27] Williams AB, Bartram CI, Modhwadia D et al. Endocoil magnetic resonance imaging quantification of external sphincter atrophy. Br J Surg 2001; 88:853-859.

[28] Fielding JR Practical MR imaging of female pelvic floor weakness. Radiographics 2002; 22:295-304.

[29] Summers HY, Hussain HK, Guire KE et al. Levator plate angle in women with pelvic organ prolapse compared to women with normal support using dynamic MR imaging. Am J Obstet Gynecol 2006; 194(5): 1427-1433.

[30] Stoker J, Zbar AP. Magnetic resonance imaging of anatomic defects in fecal incontinence. In Pescatori M, Regedas FSP, Regedas SMM, Zbar AP (eds). Imaging atlas of the pelvic floor and anorectal disease Springer-Verlag Italia, 2008; 7:39-48.

[31] Kuijpers JHC. Fecal incontinence and the anorectal angle. Neth J Surg 1984; 36:20-30.

[32] Ferrante SL, Perry RE, Schreiman JS et al. The reproducibility of measuring the anorectal angle in defecography. Dis Colon Rectum 1991; 34:51-55.

[33] Halligan S, et al. Prospective assessment of accuracy of endoanal MR imaging and endosonography in patients with fecal incontinence. AJR 2000; 175:741-745.

[34] Terra MP, Deutekom M, Beets-Tan RG et al. Relationship between external anal sphincter atrophy at endoanal magnetic resonance imaging and clinical, functional and anatomic characteristics in patients with fecal incontinence. Dis Colon Rectum, 2006; 49:668-678.

[35] Karkowski J, Pollock WF, Landon CW. Imperforate anus. Eighteen to thirty years follow-up study. Am J Surg 1973; 126:141-147.

[36] Piloni VL, Asteria CR, Bellarosa R. Defecography. In Zbar AP, Madoff RD, Wexner SD (eds). Reconstructive surgery of the Rectum, Anus and Perineum. Springer. London 2013; 2:13-20.

[37] Jen-Kou L. Preservation of anal sphincter function after hemorrhoidectomy under local anesthesia. Chin M J 2001; 64:519-524.

[38] Ihre T. Studies on anal function in continent and incontinent patients. Scand J Gastroenterol Suppl 1974; 25:1-64.

[39] Fynes MM, Behan M, O'Herlihy C et al. Anal vector volume analysis complements endoanal ultrasonographic assessment of postpartum anal sphincter injury. Br. J Surg 2000; 87:1209-1214.

[40] Samarasekera DN, Wright Y, Lowndes RH et al. Comparison of vector symmetry index and endoanal ultrasonography in the diagnosis of anal sphincter disruption. Tech Coloproctol. 2008; 12:211-215.

[41] Zbar AP, Kmiot WA, Aslam M et al. Use of vector volume manometry and endoanal magnetic resonance imaging in the adult female for assessment of anal sphincter dysfunction. Dis Colon Rectum 1999; 42:1411-1418.

[42] Podnar S. Electrodiagnosis of the anorectum: a review of techniques and clinical applications. Tech Coloproctol 2003; 7:71-76.

[43] Filler AG. Diagnosis and management of pudendal nerve entrapment syndromes: impact of MR neurography and open MR-guided injections. Neurosurg Q 2008; 18:1-6.

Chapter 6

The Evaluation of Anorectal Dysfunction in Paediatric Faecal Incontinence

Anthony G Catto-Smith and Caroline M Coffey

Additional information is available at the end of the chapter

http://dx.doi.org/10.5772/57536

1. Introduction

Voluntary control of continence and defaecation is achieved during the first few years of development in children. Its acquisition can be delayed or sometimes secondarily lost through variations in the progression of developmental maturation, but also as a consequence of organic disease and dysfunction. The psychological impact of faecal incontinence can be devastating and yet it can be extremely difficult to treat effectively.

Although many factors are critical in the maintenance of continence, the anorectum is a remarkably complex organ which is the ultimate gate-keeper, mediating sensation of rectal content and allowing selective passage or retention of gas, liquid and solids. Functional anorectal disturbances which may lead to incontinence are mediated through sensory or motor nerves, smooth or striated muscle, the physical characteristics of the anorectum, or their conscious or unconscious coordination. The evaluation of anorectal function is an important component in the assessment of faecal incontinence at any age. There are a number of modalities available for the assessment of anorectal structure and function.[1] This review will review the role of methodologies for the evaluation of anorectal function with an emphasis on paediatric faecal incontinence.

2. Methodologies for the evaluation of anorectal function

The ideal functional assessment of continence would "provide dynamic information about the integrated function of each component, mimic situations where continence is threatened, discriminate between different treatment options and not interfere unduly with the normal physiological function of the organ."[2] With these aims in view the most commonly used techniques are described.

3. Anal tone and the pull-through technique

Anal sphincter tone can be measured by the pull-through of a sphere [3] or a balloon [4] by measuring the force required to pull it rapidly past the resting or consciously squeezing anal sphincter. Wald et al found that the force required to withdraw a solid sphere was similar in controls and children with encopresis.[3]

Shandling described using a balloon inflated with saline after insertion into the rectal ampulla. The maximum force resisting the rapid pulling out of the balloon is measured by a transducer. The proposed advantage of using a balloon in preference to a solid sphere was that there less likely to be an artefactual response by the sphincters after being stretched in order to insert the device. Meunier et al found that constipated children in general had significantly increased anal tone, but only one third (19/59) of the sub-group with encopresis showed elevation and this mean was not significantly different from that of control children.[5] In a later study of constipated children (44/63 with associated encopresis), the mean anal pressure was not significantly different from controls although 38% showed values greater than the normal range.[6] Loening-Baucke observed that rapid pull-through pressure was significantly lower in a group of 20 children with encopresis when compared with matched controls.[7] Moreover this failed to improve after successful laxative treatment. These pull-through techniques are now mainly of historical interest.

4. Saline continence

Threshold of incontinence to rectally infused saline can be used to measure the overall capacity of the anorectal unit in maintaining continence during conditions which partially simulate diarrhea.[8] The threshold volume at which leakage of at least 15 mL occurs is identified. Normally, in adult practice, the total volume retained is normally factored in as well. Most adults can retain 800 mL without leakage, but normal values for children have not been established. However, encopresis usually involves incontinence to solid stool and this method may be misleading.[4] Nevertheless, it continues to be used occasionally in adults where it can provide a useful measure.[9] It is of little value in paediatric practice.

5. Balloon expulsion

Expulsion of a rectal balloon, simulating defaecation, is used as an indication of the effectiveness of the defaecation mechanism and as a training device. A balloon attached to a narrow gauge probe terminating in a 3-way stopcock is inserted into the rectum and then inflated with

http://dx.doi.org/10.5772/57536

a fluid such as water, either to a predefined volume (30-100 mL), or to sensory awareness.[8, 10, 11] The subject is asked to defaecate this within a prescribed time either seated on a toilet or in the left lateral position. Inability to evacuate the balloon within the specified time suggests the presence of anismus or dyssynergia.[8, 12] The technique may be modified by progressively reducing the distending volume in order to establish the volume at which evacuation does occur. This is generally a relatively well-accepted technique in children.

While saline continence testing and balloon expulsion provide simple screening tests for defaecatory disorders, they do not establish mechanisms.[13] They can however be used as repeated measures to define clinical progress.

6. Anorectal manometry

Manometric evaluation is the most established and widely available investigative tool for the evaluation of anorectal function.[1] It is widely used in paediatric practice, but generally requires a degree of cooperation and its utility may be limited, especially under the age of 5-6 years. Normal values obtained for children show a considerable variation depending on the technique (table 1).

Ref	N	% M	mean age (range)	ARM type	anal verge to balloon (cm)	rapid pull-through (mmHg)	resting anal tone (mmHg)	max. squeeze (mmHg)	RAIR (mL air)	transient sens'n (mL air)	prolonged sens'n (mL air)	total anal relax'n (mL air)	saline continence (mL)	balloon defaecation 100mL	anismus
[7]	20	75	8.6 (4-12y)	SS	11	133 (14)*	53 (12)	190 (49)	14 (5)						
[24]	15	66	8.5 (5- 12y)	SS	11				17 (7)	19 (7)	118 (29)	122 (46)+			
[43, 54]	16	69	10.3 (7-13y)	SS	11		67 (12)	140 (52)	11 (5)	14 (7)	101 (39)	104 (49)+	212 (47)	100%	0
[5]	32	41	8.2 (1-15y)	WP	7-15				17 (7.2)	17 (7.1)					
[6]	51	59	(4-14y)	WP	7-15	53 (9.7)**			median 15	median 20					
[55]	25	48	5.7 (2m-12y)	WP	7	median 56**	52 (7.1)		12 (4.0)						
[3]	21	52	9.6 (7-14y)	TB	5			81 (6.6)	24 (2.4)	14 (1.9)					2 (10%)
[22]	11	55	(7m-16y)	TB	7		29 (7.9)		22 (10.6)	32 (11.9)					

1 Figures: mean (SD). N=number in study, M=male. ARM=anorectal manometry. SS=solid state, WP=water perfused, TB=three balloon Pressure converted to mmHg where appropriate.

* anal resting tone=trough pressure at the maximum tone on rapid pull through-atmospheric pressure.

**anal resting tone=maximum rectal pressure-maximum anal pressure on rapid pull through.

RAIR=rectoanal inhibitory reflex

+If threshold not attained before prolonged sensation then it was deemed to have occurred at the next volume increment

Table 1. Anorectal manometric values in normal children.

Anorectal manometry can be used to define sphincter function, rectoanal reflexes, rectal sensation, rectal compliance and dynamic disorders of defaecation.

A manometric system includes four components – a pressure sensing device (probe), an amplifier or recorder for processing and storing signals, a display, and in more modern systems, software for data analysis. A variety of probes are available – these include solid state transducers, water perfused or sleeve catheters, and water or air filled balloon catheters.[8, 14] All catheters usually have a distensible end balloon. The three balloon system initially developed by Schuster [15] is not in common use in children.

The catheters are generally introduced with the patient in the left lateral position with hips and knees flexed without formal rectal preparation in the case of normal subjects, although they should be asked to empty their bowels prior to the test. No bowel preparation at all is required for very small children.[16] In the case of constipated or incontinent patients, it is advisable to wait at least 1 hour after disimpaction. The use of enemas for this procedure has been shown not to affect colonic motility or manometric parameters in healthy children[17] but it has been suggested that measurements recorded with an inadequately emptied rectum may be unreliable.[3] A digital rectal examination is always advisable to determine residual stool content and anatomy. Children who are unable to tolerate a digital rectal examination are most unlikely to accept catheter insertion.

In the case of either perfused catheters or those with transducers, pressure is measured at radially orientated directions around and/or along the catheter. Older methodologies involved distances of up to several centimeters between side-holes or transducers, but the recent move toward high definition manometry has resulted in the use of up to several pressure measuring points every centimeter. Typically, the measuring points at the extremes of the array are used to define "rectal" or abdominal pressure, and a pressure in air outside the patient. Within the array, closely spaced measuring points define the anal canal and sphincters, with overlap to allow for sphincteric movement.

There are advantages and disadvantages in each of the two systems – either water perfused or solid state transducer. Water perfused systems are cheaper, more robust, but suffer from the difficulties associated with water leakage. Solid state systems are much more accurate and convenient but also much more expensive and fragile. The physical presence of either catheter in the anal canal of this device must inevitably result in some degree of artefact, and this may be influenced by the diameter of the probe. Water leakage may also make simultaneous electromyographic (EMG) measurement using surface electrodes difficult. Both systems also suffer from the trade-off between obtaining radially-directed and longitudinal measurements at the same time. Fixed techniques without some sort of slow-station withdrawal may not accurately reflect asymmetric abnormalities in sphincteric pressure.

An estimation of the length of the anal canal and of anal resting and maximal squeeze pressure using the station or pull-through technique can be obtained by either manometric system.

Anal pressures obtained from station techniques are less than half those obtained by the rapid pull-through method, possibly due to sphincteric spasm.[7] The station method is generally preferred.[1] Anal pressures have been shown to vary significantly within individuals due to various cyclic activities.[18, 19] Age is also likely to have a substantial impact, especially in childhood. Cyclic variations in anal pressure may well be of importance in influencing propensity for soiling[20], but are practically difficult to measure in children and are not routinely measured in adults.

It has been suggested that anal hypertonia in constipated children may contribute to obstructed defaecation. Hypotonia was suggested as contributing to incontinence. Arhan et al compared resting anal and rectal pressure between constipated children (121/176 with encopresis) and a control group.[21] The mean internal anal sphincter and rectal tone pressures were significantly elevated in constipated children, but mean external anal sphincter tone was normal. Molnar subsequently similarly found that the anal canal tone was hypertonic in a group of constipated children (28/32=88% with associated soiling).[22] However, in contrast, using the station pull-through method, anal tone was found to be significantly reduced in chronically constipated children (96% with faecal incontinence) by Loening-Baucke et al.[23] This was observed to normalize in the children who recovered from constipation and soiling after treatment with laxatives as opposed to the rapid pull-through pressure which did not. [7]

Rectal filling during anorectal manometry is mimicked by the inflation of a balloon into the rectal medulla, generally with its distal point of attachment to the probe between 6 and 11cm from the anal verge. This can be used to determine the presence of the rectoanal inhibitory reflex (RAIR), define rectal sensation and as a measure of rectal compliance.[8]

Balloon distension is relatively simple to use in children, and allows an indication of internal anal sphincter, external anal sphincter (EAS), rectal and balloon pressures at rest, during voluntary squeeze and strain and rectoanal inhibitory reflex. Transient and stepwise inflation of the balloon in predetermined increments of between 5 and 30 ml allows the approximate measurement of threshold volumes of the reflex internal anal sphincter relaxation, compensatory EAS contraction, transient sensation, sensation of fullness and desire to defaecate. Normal values for these have been defined for children. Unfortunately, there are a number of differing protocols for rectal distension, each with implications for normal values which results in difficulties comparing the results from different investigators.(table 1)

The rectal sensory threshold can be difficult to define, as the duration of initial sensation on progressive stepped balloon filling tends to be very transient. As the balloon is progressively filled in a stepwise fashion, sensation becomes more and more prolonged and accompanied by a desire to defaecate. We have used sensation lasting longer than 30 seconds to define the rectal sensory threshold but find it difficult to help children distinguish between a sensory threshold and desire to defaecate. Loening-Baucke [24] suggested a minimum of 30 seconds for urge to defaecate and tried to distinguish between a sensation of fullness (or mild urgency) and also from transient sensation. Sun et al [25] distinguished between sensation of wind and a desire to defaecate. These sensations are obviously subjective and very hard to define for children.

The rectal sensory threshold appears to be elevated in children with constipation with or without associated soiling.[5, 6, 10, 22]. The threshold for sustained internal anal sphincter relaxation may occur before that of sensation.[22] This is clearly important in relation to the occurrence of faecal incontinence.

Using progressive stepwise balloon distension to identify the threshold for prolonged (30sec) urge to defaecate, Loening-Baucke found that children with faecal retention and soiling had a significant impairment in sensory thresholds.[10, 24, 26] This impairment persisted for up to

3 years in most (5 of 8) children despite apparent recovery from constipation and soiling after treatment with laxatives.[24]

The rectoanal inhibitory reflex (RAIR) is a relaxation of the internal anal sphincter occurring after distension of the rectum. Normally simultaneous contraction of the EAS and puborectalis muscle counters this and preserves continence. The reflex is absent in both Hirschsprung disease and anal achalasia.[14] There are some studies that would suggest that the distending threshold volume required to elicit this reflex is elevated in children with encopresis.

Meunier et al [5] found that the threshold for RAIR threshold was higher in 6% of constipated patients. Molnar et al [22] observed that 16% of constipated children (28/32=88% with associated soiling) had an elevated threshold. Neither value was significantly different from the control groups. Wald et al found that the threshold volume for eliciting the RAIR in encopretic children was not significantly different from that of controls.[3] This was confirmed by Loening-Baucke and Younoszai [23] in chronically constipated children (67/70 of whom soiled), although they also found that a given increase in rectal balloon volume produced a significantly smaller IAS relaxation in these children. This impaired relaxation persisted after treatment with laxatives regardless of outcome.[7] However, in a later study Loening-Baucke found a significantly elevated mean RAIR threshold in 97 constipated and encopretic children. [27] She expressed caution in interpretation of this result as the comparison control group had a lower threshold than that observed in a previous control group (see Table 1).

Over all it seems likely that at least some encopretic children do have an elevated RAIR threshold but this but this may relate to pre-existing rectal enlargement that increases the balloon distension required before the wall is stretched.

Squeeze pressures may be measured. It is useful to ask children to either "squeeze" or "strain" during manometric examination. This helps define anismus or dyssynergia. The usefulness of the actual resulting pressure value is less clear. Maximum squeeze pressure in children with encopresis was found by Wald [3] to be higher than in normal children, but not significantly so, and by Loening-Bauke [7] to be significantly lower.

Rectal compliance can be measured by intra-balloon pressures obtained during progressive, intermittent distension of a rectal balloon and comparing this with intra-balloon measured pressure during distension in air outside the patient. This provides a measure of the accommodation of the rectal wall which in turn depends on the visco-elastic properties of the wall and mobility of the adjacent viscera. Rectal compliance is decreased with age and inflammation of the rectum. A higher rectal compliance has been described in megarectum and faecal impaction. Urge incontinence may be related to reduced compliance.[28] Disturbed rectal compliance appears to be an important component of paediatric constipation, and does not seem to contribute to non-retentive faecal soiling.[29] Despite this, recovery from functional constipation in children and adolescents does not seem to be related to degree of abnormality in compliance.[30]

Balloon expulsion, though described previously, also forms part of the anorectal manometric study and can be combined with sphincter pressure measurements.

Constipated children with encopresis are significantly more likely to have difficulty defaecating a water filled balloon and produce higher and more protracted elevations in intra-abdominal pressure than controls.[26, 27] There was no apparent distinction in these small studies between the patients able and unable to defaecate the balloons either clinically or in thresholds for RAIR, transient sensation and desire to defaecate, or with the accompanying increase in abdominal pressure. Children who are able to defaecate a balloon during the manometric study are significantly more likely to recover from constipation and soiling with laxative treatment than those who could not, and the difficulty evacuating a balloon does not appear to improve with treatment. Paradoxically, some children and adults have greater difficulty with smaller balloons than larger ones.[10, 31]

Robinson and Gibbons first identified paradoxical contraction of the anal sphincters (anismus) during attempted defaecation in children with encopresis.[32] This was present in 74% of children with constipation and in none in their control group. Subsequently, paradoxical contraction has been shown to coincide with an increase in EMG during straining in contrast with control children, who showed a reduction in EMG activity.[26] There is a strong association between anismus and the inability to defaecate balloons but none with the magnitude of the increase in abdominal pressure during straining.[26] Laxative therapy was not observed to improve anismus even when remission from constipation and soiling was achieved. Children with abnormal expulsion dynamics were more likely to have primary than secondary encopresis and more severe constipation (as evidenced by a palpable faecal mass in the abdomen). The three factors of severity of constipation, anismus and inability to defaecate a 100 ml balloon were found to be predictors of laxative treatment failure.[27] Recovery has been found to be more likely in children who were trained to relax the EAS during defaecation attempts than those who did not learn to do so. In those children who learnt to relax the EAS, 100ml balloon defaecation and transient sensation threshold improved in those who recovered from constipation and soiling but not in those who did not recover.[33, 34]

Megarectum is a term which has been used indiscriminately historically to describe significant rectal distension. For various reasons, the term "enlarged rectum" is better-used for those patients with a rectum which occupies greater than 0.61 of the recto-pelvic ratio. "Megarectum" should be limited to those in whom a significant abnormality is defined on anorectal manometry, pressure-volume curves, or rectal compliance investigations.[35]

Although anorectal manometry may be regarded as socially unpleasant and invasive, in general terms it is a low risk procedure. Colonic perforation has been described,[36] and clearly the procedure should ideally be carried out gently, with a cooperative patient, appropriately stopping if significant discomfort occurs.

Most children with encopresis have some form of manometric abnormality. Meunier[6] observed that 94% of their sample of constipated children, 70% of whom had associated soiling, had an enlarged rectum when compared with normal children and 97% of these children demonstrated some form of pathophysiology.

7. Ambulatory anal manometry

This provides a method for identifying spontaneous relaxations of the anal canal during prolonged more normal physiological activity.[37] A system of non-perfused microtransducers within a probe connected to a small portable recording box is inserted into the anal canal and rectum of the subject. A marker and diary enables the identification of manometric changes coinciding with events such as the feeling of urgency, sensation of or the passage of flatus, micturition, defaecation, sleep and postural changes. Parameters of motility can be compared directly but especially over time. Recording in the upright position is more natural than in the lateral position required by conventional manometry both from a physiological and a psychological viewpoint. This recording method is in its infancy and has yet to be reported with children. It does, however, potentially provide insights into periodic variations in rectal motor activity and variations in anal tone that might explain such conditions as nocturnal incontinence and proctalgia fugax.[38, 39]

It has been found that up to one third of children with retention and/or soiling are unable to perceive rectal dilation until IAS relaxation is well established.[22] This means that these children would have difficulty maintaining continence as the rectum fills. Knowing that multiple spontaneous IAS relaxations occur during the course of a day, each of these pose a threat to continence if, in the case of a child with chronic retention, the rectum is not empty, there is no compensatory contraction of the EAS and puborectalis. and the EAS response is inadequate.[40] Failure of compensatory contraction has been identified in adults with soiling.[40] This seems likely to be the basis of "overflow" soiling which is diagnosed in children.

8. Electromyography

Electromyographic (EMG) recording of electrical activity in the external anal sphincter can give a more accurate indication of tonic activity of this sphincter than interpretation of pressure differentials from anorectal manometry, particularly when the two sphincters are working in opposition. Two types of electrodes are in predominant use: 1) surface electrodes placed near the anal verge with the reference electrode on the thigh and 2) bipolar needle electrodes inserted into the striated muscle of the sphincter. Sponge electrodes, and a solid plug electrode (both placed within the canal) have also been employed. The needle electrode causes significant discomfort and only picks up signals from adjacent motor units. It is of limited clinical value in childhood encopresis. It is certainly not appropriate for use in the conscious child. Surface electrodes are much easier to use by comparison. One criticism of surface electrodes is that they not distinguish between external anal sphincter muscular activity and that of the abductor and glutei.[41] More recent modifications using multi-electrode arrays on a gloved index finger allow the extraction of information on innervation zones position and overlapping of motor unit branches of the puborectalis muscle and its electrophysiological properties.[42] This offers considerable advantage to a paediatric population.

Sphincteric EMG activity should reduce during straining, and increase during squeezing. When recording EMG activity during strain, the accompanying increase in intra-abdominal pressure should also be confirmed. A change of less than 25% in the baseline EMG is considered normal, while an increase in activity of greater than 25% is considered to indicate incorrect defaecation dynamics or dyssynergia [27, 43]. During voluntary squeeze the increase in electric impulse activity of the EMG should be not be accompanied by an increase in abdominal pressure.

9. Radiography

Plain abdominal radiography has been suggested as a tool to assess faecal retention in children and Barr et al developed a scale for this purpose.[44] Other scales have also been developed and although they tend to have good intra-observer correlation, they generally have poor inter-observer reproducibility.[45] Meunier et al using barium enema studies observed that almost all children complaining of constipation show radiological evidence of an enlarged rectum and bowel and so considered this procedure neither diagnostic nor contributory towards an understanding of its pathophysiology.[6]

10. Gastrointestinal transit time

Gastrointestinal transit time can be assessed by measuring the rate of movement of either a single group or sequentially ingested radiopaque markers through the intestine by either a single,[46] alternate daily or daily abdominal radiographs and/or their excretion by counting them in faeces.[47-49] Cruder measurements involve the mouth to evacuation time of solid recognizable foodstuffs or colored material.[50] One modification of this technique is the radionuclide transit study, which allows a better determination of sequential progress through the entire gastrointestinal tract,[51] and more recently the wireless motility capsule.[48] Importantly, radio-opaque markers, nuclear transit and wireless capsules all provide a measure of anorectal retention.

11. Anorectal biopsy

Although Hirschsprung's disease is normally diagnosed in infancy, the possibility that a child suffering from intractable constipation with or without soiling may have this disease should be considered.[52] If it is suspected, suction rectal biopsy should be undertaken to establish the absence of ganglion cells, the universally accepted standard to confirm the diagnosis of Hirschsprung disease.

Typically, the recto-anal inhibitory reflex is absent in patients with Hirschsprung disease. Failure to wait for resting conditions to become established, using inadequate balloon volumes and interference in the tracing of the IAS by contraction of the EAS can all lead to false positive diagnosis but it has been shown to have a sensitivity of 85% and a specificity of 100%.[53]

Anorectal manometry can play a role as a screening test for children especially over the age of a year, and guide assessment in patients with Hirschsprung disease who have had surgery. It can also assist management in those in whom sphincter myectomy or botulinum toxin are being considered.[14]

12. Conclusion

A number of methods exist for the evaluation of physiological function and dysfunction in the anorectum. Anorectal manometric testing is central but the others are also key. Despite the many tests available, there is still relatively poor understanding of normal function, and especially so in children.

Abbreviations

EAS	external anal sphincter
EMG	electromyography
IAS	internal anal sphincter
RAIR	rectoanal inhibitory reflex

Author details

Anthony G Catto-Smith[1,2] and Caroline M Coffey[1]

*Address all correspondence to: tony.cattosmith@rch.org.au

1 Department of Gastroenterology, The Royal Children's Hospital, Melbourne, Australia

2 Department of Paediatrics, University of Melbourne, Australia

References

[1] Scott SM, Gladman MA. Manometric, sensorimotor and neurophysiologic evaluation of anorectal function. Gastroenterol Clin North Am. 2008;37:511-538

[2] Read NW. Functional assessment of the anorectum in faecal incontinence. In: Bock G, Whelan J, eds. Neurobiology of Incontinence: Ciba Foundation; 1990:119-138

[3] Wald A, Chandra R, Chiponis D, et al. Anorectal function and continence mechanisms in childhood encopresis. J Pediatr Gastroenterol Nutr. 1986;5:346-351

[4] Shandling B, Gilmour RF. The anal sphincter force in health and disease. J Pediatr Surg. 1987;22:754-757

[5] Meunier P, Marechal JM, de Beaujeu MJ. Rectoanal pressures and rectal sensitivity studies in chronic childhood constipation. Gastroenterology. 1979;77:330-336

[6] Meunier P, Louis D, Jaubert de Beaujeu M. Physiologic investigation of primary chronic constipation in children: comparison with the barium enema study. Gastroenterology. 1984;87:1351-1357

[7] Loening-Baucke V. Abnormal rectoanal function in children recovered from chronic constipation and encopresis. Gastroenterology. 1984;87:1299-1304

[8] Tantiphlachiva K, Rao SSC. Anorectal Manometry. In: Parkman HP, McCallum RW, Rao SSC, eds. GI Motility. Thorofare, New Jersey: Slack Incorporated; 2011:163-178

[9] Ozturk R, Niazi S, Stessman M, et al. Long-term outcome and objective changes of anorectal function after biofeedback therapy for faecal incontinence. Aliment Pharmacol Ther. 2004;20:667-674

[10] Loening-Baucke V. Factors determining outcome in children with chronic constipation and faecal soiling. Gut. 1989;30:999-1006

[11] Kawimbe BM, Papachrysostomou M, Binnie NR, et al. Outlet obstruction constipation (anismus) managed by biofeedback. Gut. 1991;32:1175-1179

[12] Azpiroz F, Enck P, Whitehead WE. Anorectal functional testing: review of collective experience. Am J Gastroenterol. 2002;97:232-240

[13] Bove A, Pucciani F, Bellini M, et al. Consensus statement AIGO/SICCR: diagnosis and treatment of chronic constipation and obstructed defecation (part I: diagnosis). World Journal of Gastroenterology. 2012;18:1555-1564

[14] Le-Carlson M, Berquist W. Anorectal manometry. In: Faure C, Di Lorenzo C, Thapar N, eds. Pediatric Neurogastroenterology. New York: Humana Press; 2013:119-128

[15] Schuster MM, Hendrix TR, Mendeloff AI. The internal anal sphincter response: manometric studies on its normal physiology, neural pathways, and alteration in bowel disorders. J Clin Invest. 1963;42:196-207

[16] Di Lorenzo C, Hillemeier C, Hyman P, et al. Manometry studies in children: minimum standards for procedures. Neurogastroenterol Motil. 2002;14:411-420

[17] Loening-Baucke V, Younoszai MK. Effect of treatment on rectal and sigmoid motility in chronically constipated children. Pediatrics. 1984;73:199-205

[18] Enck P, Eggers E, Koletzko S, et al. Spontaneous variation of anal "resting" pressure in healthy humans. Am J Physiol. 1991;261:G823-826

[19] Sun WM, Read NW. Anorectal function in normal human subjects: effect of gender. Int J Colorectal Dis. 1989;4:188-196

[20] Sun WM, Katsinelos P, Horowitz M, et al. Disturbances in anorectal function in patients with diabetes mellitus and faecal incontinence. Eur J Gastroenterol Hepatol. 1996;8:1007-1012

[21] Arhan P, Devroede G, Jehannin B, et al. Idiopathic disorders of fecal continence in children. Pediatrics. 1983;71:774-779

[22] Molnar D, Taitz LS, Urwin OM, et al. Anorectal manometry results in defecation disorders. Arch Dis Child. 1983;58:257-261

[23] Loening-Baucke V, Younoszai MK. Abnormal and sphincter response in chronically constipated children. J Pediatr. 1982;100:213-218

[24] Loening-Baucke V. Sensitivity of the sigmoid colon and rectum in children treated for chronic constipation. J Pediatr Gastroenterol Nutr. 1984;3:454-459

[25] Sun WM, Read NW, Prior A, et al. Sensory and motor responses to rectal distention vary according to rate and pattern of balloon inflation. Gastroenterology. 1990;99:1008-1015

[26] Loening-Baucke V, Cruikshank BM. Abnormal defecation dynamics in chronically constipated children with encopresis. J Pediatr. 1986;108:562-566

[27] Loening-Baucke V. Factors responsible for persistence of childhood constipation. J Pediatr Gastroenterol Nutr. 1987;6:915-922

[28] Chan CL, Lunniss PJ, Wang D, et al. Rectal sensorimotor dysfunction in patients with urge faecal incontinence: evidence from prolonged manometric studies. Gut. 2005;54:1263-1272

[29] Voskuijl WP, van Ginkel R, Benninga MA, et al. New insight into rectal function in pediatric defecation disorders: disturbed rectal compliance is an essential mechanism in pediatric constipation. J Pediatr. 2006;148:62-67

[30] van den Berg MM, Voskuijl WP, Boeckxstaens GE, et al. Rectal compliance and rectal sensation in constipated adolescents, recovered adolescents and healthy volunteers. Gut. 2008;57:599-603

[31] Lestar B, Penninckx F, Kerremans R. Biofeedback defaecation training for anismus. Int J Colorectal Dis. 1991;6:202-207

[32] Robinson BA, Gibbons JSE. Paradoxical external anal sphincter function in fecal retention with soiling, and its operant conditioning (abstract). Gastroenterology. 1976;70

[33] Loening-Baucke V. Efficacy of biofeedback training in improving faecal incontinence and anorectal physiologic function. Gut. 1990;31:1395-1402

[34] Loening-Baucke V. Persistence of chronic constipation in children after biofeedback treatment. Dig Dis Sci. 1991;36:153-160

[35] van der Plas RN, Benninga MA, Staalman CR, et al. Megarectum in constipation. Arch Dis Child. 2000;83:52-58

[36] Cho YB, Lee WY, Yun HR, et al. Colonic perforation caused by anorectal manometry. Int J Colorectal Dis. 2008;23:219-220

[37] Ronholt C, Rasmussen OO, Christiansen J. Ambulatory manometric recording of anorectal activity. Dis Colon Rectum. 1999;42:1551-1559

[38] Rao SS, Hatfield RA. Paroxysmal anal hyperkinesis: a characteristic feature of proctalgia fugax. Gut. 1996;39:609-612

[39] Rao SS, Welcher K. Periodic rectal motor activity: the intrinsic colonic gatekeeper? Am J Gastroenterol. 1996;91:890-897

[40] Sun WM, Donnelly TC, Read NW. Utility of a combined test of anorectal manometry, electromyography, and sensation in determining the mechanism of 'idiopathic' faecal incontinence. Gut. 1992;33:807-813

[41] Speakman CT, Henry MM. The work of an anorectal physiology laboratory. Baillieres Clin Gastroenterol. 1992;6:59-73

[42] Cescon C, Bottin A, Fernandez Fraga XL, et al. Detection of individual motor units of the puborectalis muscle by non-invasive EMG electrode arrays. J Electromyogr Kinesiol. 2008;18:382-389

[43] Loening-Baucke V. Modulation of abnormal defecation dynamics by biofeedback treatment in chronically constipated children with encopresis. J Pediatr. 1990;116:214-222

[44] Barr RG, Levine MD, Wilkinson RH, et al. Chronic and occult stool retention: a clinical tool for its evaluation in school-aged children. Clin Pediatr (Phila). 1979;18:674, 676, 677-679, passim

[45] Pensabene L, Buonomo C, Fishman L, et al. Lack of utility of abdominal x-rays in the evaluation of children with constipation: comparison of different scoring methods. J Pediatr Gastroenterol Nutr. 2010;51:155-159

[46] Bautista Casasnovas A, Varela Cives R, Villanueva Jeremias A, et al. Measurement of colonic transit time in children. J Pediatr Gastroenterol Nutr. 1991;13:42-45

[47] Cummings JH, Wiggins HS. Transit through the gut measured by analysis of a single stool. Gut. 1976;17:219-223

[48] Rao SS, Camilleri M, Hasler WL, et al. Evaluation of gastrointestinal transit in clinical practice: position paper of the American and European Neurogastroenterology and Motility Societies. Neurogastroenterol Motil. 2011;23:8-23

[49] Wald A. Colonic and anorectal motility testing in clinical practice. Am J Gastroenterol. 1994;89:2109-2115

[50] Becker U, Elsborg L. A new method for the determination of gastrointestinal transit times. Scand J Gastroenterol. 1979;14:355-359

[51] Southwell BR, Clarke MC, Sutcliffe J, et al. Colonic transit studies: normal values for adults and children with comparison of radiological and scintigraphic methods. Pediatric Surgery International. 2009;25:559-572

[52] Heuckeroth RO. Hirschsprung Disease. In: Faure C, Di Lorenzo C, Thapar N, eds. Pediatric Neurogastroenterology: Springer; 2013:271-283

[53] Aaronson I, Nixon HH. A clinical evaluation of anorectal pressure studies in the diagnosis of Hirschsprung's disease. Gut. 1972;13:138-146

[54] Loening-Baucke V, Desch L, Wolraich M. Biofeedback training for patients with myelomeningocele and fecal incontinence. Dev Med Child Neurol. 1988;30:781-790

[55] Corazziari E, Cucchiara S, Staiano A, et al. Gastrointestinal transit time, frequency of defecation, and anorectal manometry in healthy and constipated children. J Pediatr. 1985;106:379-382

Section 3

Therapy and Outcome

Chapter 7

Pelvic Floor Rehabilitation in Anal Incontinence

Claudia Regina de Souza Santos,
Tania das Graças de Souza Lima,
Fernanda Mateus Queiroz Schmidt and
Vera Lúcia Conceição de Gouveia Santos

Additional information is available at the end of the chapter

http://dx.doi.org/10.5772/57364

1. Introduction

Anal incontinence (AI) tends to be underreported to health professionals due to cultural aspects, embarrassment, mistaken perception that it is a normal consequence of aging, or because it causes little discomfort to the patient.

Maintenance of continence is essential for the normal functioning of individuals. Continence disturbances may contribute to the development of introverted behaviors, resulting in social isolation from family and friends, and may lead some people to seek help from health professionals. Elderly persons with fecal incontinence (FI) usually seek professional help or institutionalization because of precarious housing conditions, poor relationships with their partner and family members (caregivers or not), impaired cognition, presence of debilitating diseases, and financial difficulties, which seem to play a major role in their decision.

If not treated, the frequency of incontinent episodes and the amount lost increase, leading to foul odor, wet or soiled clothes, and even falls associated with fractures and death in more severe cases. Sexually active older women may fear having incontinent episodes during sexual activity, resulting in distress and sexual abstinence[1]. People only seek professional help when feeling very uncomfortable with their condition. However, health professionals may or not may be sensitive to the concerns of patients, meaning that some patients receive information and treatment while others do not.

Thus, although AI poses no immediate health risk, several studies have reported the negative impact of this condition on quality of life, leading to social isolation, concerns, decreased self-esteem and embarrassing situations [2, 3, 4, 5, 6, 7, 8, 9, 10, 11]. Besides sociocultural aspects, the Brazilian health system is based on the treatment of diseases, and actions focused on early diagnoses and prevention are still in initial stages. In the field of elderly care, the Brazilian health system has a recent National Health Policy for the Elderly, which is beginning to lead to the implementation of preventive and diagnostic measures. However, although health services for the aged have the means to assess urinary incontinence (UI) and FI, they are in small number. This can be mainly attributed to the lack of specialists, nurses, physiotherapists and physicians, resulting in reduced access to treatment for a significant portion of the population [12]. These factors certainly point to the need to increase the number of studies on the health of the elderly, which is the age group with the highest incidence of AI.

Anal incontinence has been defined in various ways, but the definition established by the International Continence Society (ICS) as "the involuntary loss of feces or flatus" is the most widely accepted [13].

Epidemiological research on AI comprises studies with different designs that have been conducted in the elderly and women, with a smaller number being conducted in the general population, people with diabetes mellitus, pregnant women, and among those with neurological disorders.

Studies have reported a high prevalence of AI of up to 33% [14], especially among women [15], beginning after childbirth and aggravating with multiple births and advanced age (above 65 years of age) [16].

In Brazil, there are few studies on AI in both general and specific populations. A study conducted in a random sample of 519 adults from the general population of a city in Minas Gerais reported a prevalence of FI of 7%, with higher prevalence rates (4%) among women1. Other study performed in a random stratified sample of 1162 adults living in the city of Londrina (Paraná) found a self-reported prevalence of AI of 3.6% (4% among women and 3% among men); with 70.1% of participants with AI reporting liquid stool incontinence. A study carried out in Porto Alegre (Rio Grande do Sul) with 1168 patients from general health services observed that 37% of patients aged 41 years and older had AI, with 44% of them being women18. In a group of 40 elderly persons participating in a program for the improvement of daily living and instrumental activities, only one of them (2.5%) had FI19. Another study reported prevalence rates of 2% for solid stool incontinence, 15% for liquid stool incontinence, and 27% for flatus incontinence in 100 postmenopausal women aged 45 years or older20.

Few studies on this field with varying prevalence rates are found in the international literature. A study conducted in a random sample of 4277 elderly persons of both sexes, aged 75 years and older found a prevalence of FI of 16.9%, increasing with age [21]. A second study reported a prevalence of FI of 12%, with men having higher rates (12.4%) than women (11.6%) [22]. In a recent survey performed in Taiwan with people aged 65 year and older, 6.9% of 1345 men and 9.3% of 1370 women reported having FI23. In patients from gastroenterology and gynecology clinics in Switzerland, AI was more prevalent among women (7.5%) [24]. A prevalence of FI higher than 55% was found among women attending gynecology clinics and a local family planning clinic in the UK [25]. A lower prevalence of FI (10.4%) was observed in a sample of 4815 women aged from 82 to87 years living in Australia [26].

The most cited risk-factors or predictors associated with AI are female gender [15, 24, 25], advanced age [16], perineal and surgical lesions combined with a feeling of incomplete defecation [27], multiple births [28], and anorectal and urogynecologic surgeries [17]. In addition, other authors have also cited idiopathic factors, rectal prolapse, menopause, and traumas [29]; diarrhea whether infectious or not [17]; inflammatory bowel disease combined with abusive use of laxatives, fecal impaction, rectal neoplasia and neuropathy [30]; immobility and dementia [31]; neurological diseases and disorders such as multiple sclerosis and Parkinson disease [17]; fistulotomy and ileal pouch reconstruction [8]; and median episiotomy [31, 14].

The association of diabetes with AI, especially among the elderly, is worthy of note. In a group of 113 elderly persons, who were receiving outpatient follow-up, 2.4% of them reported having AI at least 5 years after diabetes diagnosis [32]. Diabetes was one of the factors associated with AI in a group of 4815 women aged 82-87 years [26]. The effects of hyperglycemia on anorectal motor and sensory function was assessed in 18 patients with diabetes (8 with type 1 and 10 with type 2 diabetes) by a systematic measurement of blood glucose and measurements of anorectal motility and sensation. The results revealed that acute hyperglycemia inhibits external anal sphincter function and decreases rectal compliance, potentially increasing the risk of FI [33]. An experimental study with male Wistar rats suggested that high glycemic levels may cause hypotonia of the anal sphincter, which may lead to complications such as FI [34].

2. Conservative treatment of anal incontinence

Epidemiological data on AI and its impact on the quality of life of individuals indicate the need for early diagnosis and prevention of this condition. However, this is not always possible because AI tends to be underreported by patients and underinvestigated by health professionals.

Anal incontinence can usually be treated by surgical or conservative means, according to the etiology and severity of the condition, and clinical status of the patient.

In this chapter, only the conservative treatment of AI is described and discussed.

The conservative treatment consists of nutritional-hygienic interventions and perineal rehabilitation through pelvic floor muscle training (PFMT).

2.1. Nutritional-hygienic interventions (behavioral change)

Behavioral change is part of the conservative treatment, consisting of techniques that contribute to restoration of continence, especially in the presence of fecal urgency.

In these cases, where the urgency situation itself may lead to anxiety, it is recommended that the individual's ability to retain fecal matter be increased by delaying defecation, which can be achieved by training on the toilet. The individual should be instructed to seat on the toilet when feeling the urge to defecate and try to retain the passage of feces for 1 minute on the clock. The next step is to increase the contraction duration to 5 minutes and then gradually to

10 minutes. After achieving success, the training should be performed in the bedroom far from the bathroom. In this way, the person will also be working at the emotional level. The use of pelvic floor muscle exercises, as will be described, completes the treatment [35]

Among other behavioral interventions, the patient should be instructed to:

- Avoid the use of laxatives
- Have a private and comfortable place to defecate
- Try to respond to the gastrocolic reflex by defecating 15 to 30 minutes after breakfast
- Seek treatment for anorectal diseases, such as hemorrhoids, fissures and fistulas
- Improvise a support for the feet during defecation, maintaining the legs elevated when in the seating position to prevent straining
- Have a dietary fiber* intake of 6 to 10 g/day and an adequate ingestion of liquids (8 glasses of water or 1500 ml/day, increasing the intake during summer)
- Take regular exercise (if not contraindicated) [36].

* people with diabetes mellitus should have systematic monitoring due to the ingestion of carbohydrates associated with dietary fibers [36].

In addition to these guidelines, it is important for the individual to develop a sense of complete evacuation and examine the stool for the presence of uncommon substances, such as blood and mucus.

2.2. Rehabilitation of the pelvic floor

Although the role of the pelvic floor muscle in AI is not fully understood [37], it is believed that this muscle is a key factor in maintaining anal continence. Pelvic floor muscle training is the conservative treatment most commonly used in the management of pelvic floor dysfunctions [38, 39, 40, 41]. However, the lack of scientific evidence to support this therapy may limit its indication, thus reducing its chances of success [42].

2.2.1. Pelvic floor exercises

The impairment of the sphincter function is the cause of or major contributing factor to anal incontinence. Exercises for PFMT are a strategy to improve sphincter function. Although there is no consensus among various authors, many of them believe that repeated contractions of the anal sphincter and pelvic floor muscle increase the strength, duration and speed of recruitment of the external anal sphincter, and also increases the patient's ability to contract the pelvic floor muscle alone and to maintain it contracted [43, 44, 35].

Improvements in muscle tone and sphincter strength lead to an increase in the strength of the anal canal and patient's ability to delay defecation [45]. Exercises for PFMT were first described by Arnold Kegel [46] in 1948 for the treatment of UI with the objective of improving pelvic floor muscle contraction and increasing urethral closure pressure. The exercises are based on the principle that repeated voluntary contractions of the pelvic floor muscle, if correctly performed, contribute to an increase in urethral strength and resistance during muscle contraction and relaxation [47, 48].

Pelvic floor muscle exercise (PFME) programs are based on the assumption that it is possible to increase hypertrophy and aerobic and anaerobic capacity of muscles [49]. Strong and repetitive exercises increase muscle volume, and prolonged contractions of moderate intensity increase resistance and may improve resting pressure and contraction of the pelvic floor [50, 35]. Pelvic floor muscle training was introduced for the treatment of AI in the 1970s as a way to improve the results of PFME programs [51].

Although the objectives of PFME are well defined, little consensus exists among clinicians about the best exercise program. Specialists have recommended maintaining the contraction of the pelvic floor muscle between 1 to 30 seconds, with 30 to 45 repetitions per day or 1 to 50 repetitions per session. A not so recent but comprehensive work [52] (Wells, 1990) reviewed 22 studies on PFME and found protocols instructing participants to perform 15 to 160 contractions a day, holding each contraction for 2 to 30 seconds.

Moreover, there are variations in the specific exercise instructions among different authors. Some programs combine exercises for strengthening both type I and type II muscle fibers while other programs use separate sets of exercise for each type of muscle fiber [47, 53].

Sampselle and Miller (1994) [54] presented a five-level program of PFME. The first level consists of muscle identification and a series of fast contractions; the second level is involved in the improvement of muscle identification; the third and fourth levels comprise muscle strengthening exercises; and the fifth level is focused on maintaining muscle strength. For all levels, the total contraction duration of the pelvic floor muscle should range from 5 to 10 minutes a day, and from 5 to 10 minutes a week after the patient reaches the fifth level.

A panel of four specialists recommended a standardized program of up to 5 rapid contractions (type II muscle fibers) and 5 slow contractions (type I muscle fibers) to be performed 10 times a day [55] (Continence Foundation, 2000). This same protocol was used by Solomon and collaborators (2003) [56] in Australia, by Norton and Chelvanayagam (2004) [35] at the St. Mark's Hospital in London, and by health professionals at the Outpatient Biofeedback Clinic of the "Clementino Fraga Filho" University Hospital (HUCFF) in Brazil since 2006.

As in the St. Mark's Hospital (Norton e Chelvanayagam, 2001) [57], patients treated at the Outpatient Biofeedback Clinic (HUCFF) are advised to not expect immediate results from PFME. The sessions are scheduled at 2- to 4-week intervals, according to the patient understanding of the program, individual progress, and possibility of having the patient to come to the clinic for a training session. Weekly sessions are not recommended because positive results usually take 2 to 4 months to be obtained, resulting in a large number of PFME sessions before any improvement is noted, which may discourage the patient from continuing the treatment.

There is no evidence-based protocol for a PFME program; however, it should be tailored to the individual with respect to the number and duration of contractions, and number of repetitions. The instructions should be given in written form in the first session and orally reviewed during subsequent sessions.

2.2.2. Biofeedback: An important step in pelvic floor rehabilitation

Biofeedback refers to techniques that make unconscious body processes perceptible to the senses, so they can be manipulated by conscious control [35].

According to Norton and collaborators (2010) [58], there is no standardization in the literature about the use of biofeedback in the treatment of AI. These authors proposed three main training categories (strength, sensorial and coordination), which may be combined in a biofeedback program. Historically, PFMT is seldom used without biofeedback in the treatment of AI. The success of the PFMT depends on the ability of the patient to correctly perform a voluntary contraction of the pelvic floor muscle before beginning the Rehabilitation of the Pelvic Floor Program [58]. The combination of PFMT with biofeedback is also used in our daily practice.

One of the major obstacles in the re-education and rehabilitation of the pelvic floor muscle is that most patients have difficulty in correctly identifying and isolating the muscles [59]. Most women do not have the ability to recognize their pelvic floor muscle and do not know how to exercise it [60]; about 60% of women are unable to effectively contract this muscle, even when written or oral instructions are provided [35].

In order to increase muscle awareness and the ability to voluntarily contract the muscle, the patient will need to understand and find a way to control the pelvic floor muscle. This can be achieved using different approaches, with biofeedback being the best method for the treatment of AI. This technique improves symptoms in about 70% of cases by increasing the strength, duration and speed of recruitment of the external anal sphincter and the patient's ability to contract the pelvic floor muscle alone [61, 62, 63, 56, 35, 64].

For some authors, if AI is caused by damage of the pelvic floor, leading to sphincter weakness or inability to sense the presence of stool in the rectum, biofeedback is the treatment of choice, eliminating or decreasing the number of incontinence episodes, and resulting in a 90% improvement in 72% of cases [65].

Biofeedback therapy is relatively easy and safe to be performed, has no adverse effects, is well-tolerated, stimulates the patient, although it requires a specialist to conduct the program, and may be carried out using several techniques and devices.

Among the various techniques available, biofeedback by digital guidance and manometric biofeedback have been used successfully [66]. Both biofeedback programs assist the patient in perceiving muscle contraction in real time by either digital guidance and oral command or graphic visual display of the muscular contraction on a device screen, as will be described next.

2.2.2.1. Biofeedback by digital guidance, according to Solomon (2003) [56] and Doughty and Burns (2006) [59]

Patients in left lateral decubitus position with the legs flexed are instructed to contract the external anal sphincter by digital guidance and oral command. For this purpose, the index finger is inserted into the anus of the patient, who is instructed to contract the muscle upon request.

2.2.2.2. Biofeedback with anorectal manometry, according to Solomon (2003) [56]:

In this type of biofeedback, anorectal manometry is performed using a perfusion system with three or four channels to create a graphic visual display of the voluntary contraction pressure.

After application of lubricant gel, a catheter is inserted into the anal canal and coupled to a computer. The patient is then instructed to contract the external anal sphincter and observe the graphic display of the contraction on the computer screen. The graphic shows the muscle recruitment strength and duration of the voluntary muscle contraction, representing the muscle activity. At that moment, the patient is instructed on how to identify the sphincter function and to reproduce what was shown in real time on the computer screen.

This training is also performed with the patient in left lateral decubitus position and in front of the device display, so that the patient can immediately and clearly see the readings of contraction and relaxation pressures on the screen.

Several studies on biofeedback, using different methodologies, have reported improvement in objective indicators, including rest and contraction pressures, when comparing pre- and post-treatment values [67, 68, 69, 70, 71, 72]. Other studies have found positive results in subjective indicators, such as severity level of AI and quality of life [71, 9, 73] (Byrne, 2005; Yusuf, 2004; Bartlett, 2009) or in both objective and subjective indicators [56].

A non-randomized clinical trial on biofeedback combined with PFMEs was conducted in Rio de Janeiro (Brazil) with 38 patients, who were allocated to either the manometry group (n = 20) or digital guidance group (n =18). For both groups, statistically significant increases in rest pressure and contraction pressure, as well as improvement in subjective indicators were found after 8 biofeedback sessions, when comparing pre- and post-treatment values [74].

Few clinical trials on the use of biofeedback as a conservative treatment in patients with AI can be found in the international literature. Despite the fact that this technique has been widely cited, studies have not properly described both the methods and evaluation criteria used.

3. Neuromuscular electrical stimulation

The conservative treatment of AI has recently included the use of neuromuscular electrical stimulation alone or in combination with other treatments in specific conditions.

3.1. Neuromuscular electrical stimulation of the pelvic floor

Neuromuscular electrical stimulation of the pelvic floor (NMESPV) is performed by applying electrical current to the pelvic floor muscle. Electrical stimulation using an excitomotor current provides muscle strengthening, hypertrophy, increased muscle tone, and perception of motor commands, increasing the patient's ability to contract the anal canal and defecate [75]. Functional electrical stimulation activates both sensory and motor axons [76].

NMESPV is mainly applied in the treatment of sphincter dysfunction and in the stimulated gracilis neosphincter operation [75]. The procedure is performed by placing two self-adhesive transcutaneous surface electrodes on the perianal region or using endoanal probes. As technology has advanced, more comfortable surface electrodes have become available, either as skin or intra-anal plug devices with a battery box [77]. Electrical stimulation parameters, including pulse frequency, width, intensity, and on/off ratios should be properly set, because incorrect parameters may lead to fatigue and other damage [76].

The treatment is usually delivered in 2 to 3 weekly sessions, each of 20 to 40 minutes duration, varying according to the protocol, technique employed, and electrical parameters of the equipment used in the procedure. The mean length of treatment is about 3 months. At present, there is no experimental evidence upon which to select optimum electrical stimulation parameters for different symptoms and clinical conditions [76].

Contraindications for NESPV are pregnancy, use of a cardiac pacemaker, recent pelvic or abdominal surgery, hemorrhoids (in case of endo-anal electrical stimulation), radiotherapy to the pelvic region, denervation of the pelvic floor, and infection [78].

There are few studies in the literature on the application of electrical stimulation to the anal canal or perianal muscles for the treatment of FI. Electrical stimulation parameters vary among studies and the procedures are usually combined with those of other therapies.

Mergulhão (2004) [75] reported on the efficacy of anorectal neuromuscular electrical stimulation, alone or in combination with biofeedback, in the treatment of FI in multiparous women. In contrast, other authors suggested that the main effect of anorectal neuromuscular electrical stimulation is possibly not sphincter contraction, but sensitization of the patient to the anal area, or simply the effect of intervening *per se* (Mahony et al., 2004; Norton, Gibbs and Kamm, 2006) [79, 77]. Norton, Gibbs and Kamm (2006) [77] found no difference between results from electrical stimulation at 35Hz and 1Hz, and concluded that any effect may be sensory rather than direct muscle strengthening, or even a placebo effect.

A Cochrane review conducted by Hosker, Cody and Norton in 2007 [80] concluded that there was not enough evidence up to that date to judge whether electrical stimulation has a positive effect on the management of FI. Exercises and electrical stimulation may be more helpful than perineal exercises alone for women with FI after childbirth. On the other hand, a recent systematic review of 13 randomized trials on the use of feedback alone or in combination with electrical stimulation has shown that there is sufficient evidence that biofeedback combined with electrical stimulation is more efficient than biofeedback alone [81]. Thus, further studies are necessary to evaluate the use of NESPV alone or in combination of other therapies in the management of AI [80, 76].

Norton and colleagues (2009) [76] made the following recommendations for future investigations on the use electrical stimulation in the treatment of FI:

- Randomized controlled trials with adequate sample sizes are necessary to investigate all aspects of the effectiveness of electrical stimulation in FI
- The effect of electrical stimulation in changing the patient's awareness of the pelvic floor muscles is one of the interesting future areas for research

http://dx.doi.org/10.5772/57364

- A basic knowledge of electrical stimulation parameters and their likely physiological effects is essential when planning future research

3.2. Other types of electrical stimulation for the treatment of AI — Neuromodulation

3.2.1. Sacral Nerve Stimulation (SNS)

Sacral nerve stimulation (SNS) is an alternative technique for the treatment of AI. If conservative treatments fail, this is a minimally invasive technique that allows modulation of the nerves and muscles of the pelvic floor and hindgut [82, 83, 84]. SNS uses electrical stimulation applied to the sacral nerves, eliciting a physiological effect on the lower bowel, anal sphincter and pelvic floor, resulting in clinical benefit [82]. It involves inserting electrodes in the lower back and connecting them to a pulse generator. The electrical pulses affect the nerves controlling the lower part of the bowel and the anal sphincters [82, 83]. SNS application is usually safe and easy, with a limited rate of complications or adverse events. The surgical procedure is usually made under local anesthesia. Initially, a temporary lead is connected to a pulse generator outside the body. The SNS effectiveness can be reliably tested for a short period of time before the decision for a permanent implant [84]. If symptoms have improved enough, the temporary lead is replaced with a permanent one connecting the electrodes to a pulse generator implanted in the abdomen or buttock [83].

Mowatt, Glazener and Jarrett (2007) [83] conducted a Cochrane Review and concluded that there is very limited evidence suggesting that SNS can improve continence in selected people with fecal/anal incontinence. The authors also pointed out that temporary percutaneous stimulation for a two-to-three week period does not always successfully identify those for whom a permanent implant will be beneficial. Thus, good quality randomized crossover trials are needed to assess the effects of SNS on these conditions with more certainty.

3.2.2. Electrical stimulation of the posterior tibial nerve

Electrical stimulation of the posterior tibial nerve (ESPTN) has been used in the treatment of UI [85] (Schreiner, 2009) and has also been evaluated by some authors for the treatment of AI, with favorable results. ESPTN involves the reflexive stimulation of the posterior tibial nerve and may be performed by means of acupuncture, electroacupuncture, and transcutaneous electrical stimulation. It may be applied by transcutaneous electrical nerve stimulation (TENS) using electrodes placed in the region of the tibial nerve near the malleolar region. Although first described more than 20 years ago, the action mechanisms of ESPTN are not fully understood [86].

4. Final considerations

Both the academic and practical aspects of AI have been little investigated in Brazil and in the world.

In countries such as Brazil, whose population pyramid is expected to be inverted within the next 30 years due to an ever-increasing aging population, it is essential that programs for early diagnosis and prevention of chronic health conditions including incontinences and particularly AI be implemented.

Coloproctologists, wound, ostomy and continence nurses, and physiotherapists need to conduct studies to develop appropriate, cost-effective and evidence-based protocols for the treatment of AI, aimed at improving objective and subjective indicators, including quality of life.

Author details

Claudia Regina de Souza Santos[1,4,7,8], Tania das Graças de Souza Lima[6], Fernanda Mateus Queiroz Schmidt[4,5] and Vera Lúcia Conceição de Gouveia Santos[2,3,4]

1 Enterostomal Therapy Outpatient Clinic, Pouso Alegre City Public Health Department, Brasil

2 School of Nursing, University of São Paulo, Brasil

3 WCET Education Committee, Brasil

4 Brazilian Stoma Therapy Nursing Association: Ostomy, Wound and Continence Care (SOBEST), Brasil

5 Regional Cancer Hospital Santa Casa de Misericordia de Passos - Minas Gerais, Brasil

6 University Hospital Clementino Filho - Federal University of Rio de Janeiro (UFRJ), Brasil

7 World Council of Enterostomal Therapy (WCET), Brasil

8 Wound, Ostomy and Continence Nurses Society (WOCN), Brasil

References

[1] Santos CRS, Santos VLCG. Prevalence of fecal incontinence in the urban population of Pouso Alegre - Minas Gerais – Brazil. Rev Esc Enferm USP. 2011; 45(1):180-6.

[2] Johanson JF, Lafferty J. Epidemiology of fecal incontinence: the silent affliction. Am J Gastroenterol. 1996;91(1):33-6.

[3] Byrne CM, Pager CK, Rex J, Roberts R, Solomon MJ. Assessment of quality of life in the treatment of patients with neuropathic fecal incontinence. Dis Colon Rectum. 2002; 45(11):1431-6.

[4] Feldner Jr PC, Bezerra LRPS, Girão MJBC, Castro RA, Sartori MGF, Baracat EC, et al. Valor da queixa clínica e exame físico no diagnóstico da incontinência urinária. Rev Bras Ginecol Obstet. 2002; 24(2):87-91.

[5] Fuchsjager MH, Maier AG. Imaging fecal incontinence. Eur J Radiol. 2003; 47(2): 108-16.

[6] Santos VLCG, Silva AM. Qualidade de vida de pessoas com incontinência anal. Ver Bras Coloproctol. 2002; 22(2):98-108.

[7] Miner PB Jr. Economic and personal impact of fecal and urinary incontinence. Gastroenterology [serial on the internet]. 2004 [cited 2007 Aug]; 126 (suppl 1): S8-13 [about 1 p.]. Available from:

[8] Nelson RL. Epidemiology of fecal incontinence.Gastroenterology. 2004; 126: (1 Suppl 1):S3-7.

[9] Yusuf SA, Jorge JM, Habr-Gama A, Kiss DR, Gama Rodrigues J. Avaliação da qualidade de vida na incontinência anal:validação do questionário FIQL. Arq Gastroenterol. 2004;41(3):202-8.

[10] Barber MD, Walters MD, Bump RC. Short forms of two condition-specific quality-of-life questionnaires for women with pelvic floor disorders (PFDI-20 and PFIQ-7). Am J Obstet Gynecol. 2005; 193(1):103-13.

[11] Dedeli O, Fadiloglu C, Bor S. Validity and reliability of a Turkish version of the Fecal Incontinence Quality of Life Scale. J Wound Ostomy Continence Nurs. 2009; 36(5): 532-8.

[12] Bandeira EMFS, Pimenta FAP, Souza MC. Secretaria do Estado da Saúde. Atenção à saúde do idoso. Belo Horizonte: SAS/MG, 2006. 186p. Disponível em: www.saude.mg.gov.br

[13] Abrams P, Cardozo L, Khoury S, Wein A. Third Internationa Consultation on Incontinence; 2005 June 26-29; Mônaco [CD-ROM]. Monaco: International Continence Society; 2005.

[14] Montes CB, Servin JAC, Vasquez JLG. Fecal incontinence, occult lesions to the anal sphincter and related factors in primiparous patients without median routine episiotomy. Cir Ciruj. 2006; 74(6):449-55.

[15] Shiow-Shiun Horng, Yiing-Jenq Chou, Nicole Huang, Yi-Ting Fang, Pesus Chou. Fecal ncontinence epidemiology and help seeking among older people in Taiwan. Neurourology and Urodynamics. Article first published online: 2 SEP 2013.

[16] López AJG. Incontinência anal. IATREIA. 2002;15(3):190-9.

[17] Santos VLCG, Domansky RC, Hanate C, Matos DS, Benvenuto CVC, Jorge JMN. Self-reported fecal incontinence in a Community Dwelling, Urban population in Southern Brazil. JWOCN 2013 (accepted for publication).

[18] Zaslavsky C, Jurach MT, Barros CP et al. Epidemiologia da incontinência anal em população assistida em serviços de saúde de Porto Alegre/RS. Revista da AMRIGS, Porto Alegre. 2012; 56(4):289-294.

[19] Costa EC,, Nakatani AYK, Bachion MM. Capacidade de idosos da comunidade para desenvolver Atividades de Vida Diária e Atividades Instrumentais de Vida Diária. Acta Paul Enferm 2006; 19(1):43-35.

[20] Oliveira SCM, Neto AMP, Conde DM, Góes JRN, Sá DA, Paiva LC. Incontinência fecal em mulheres na pós-menopausa; prevalência, intensidade e fatores associados. Arq Gastroenterol. 2006; 43(2): 102-6.

[21] Stenzelius K, Mattiasson A, Hallberg IR, Westergren A. Symptoms of urinary and faecal incontinence among men and women 75+ in relations to health complaints and quality of life. Neurourol. Urodynam. 2000; 23: 211–222.

[22] Goode PS, Burgio KL, Halli AD,. Jones RW, Richter HE, Redden DT, Baker PS, Allman RM. Prevalence and Correlates of Fecal Incontinence in Community-Dwelling Older Adults. Journal of the American Geriatrics Society. 2005; 53(4): 629–635.

[23] Horng SS, Chou YJ, Huang N, Fang YT, Chou P. Fecal incontinence epidemiology and help seeking among older people in Taiwan. Neurourol Urodyn. 2013. Epub ahead of print.

[24] Damon H, Guye O, Seigneurin A, Long F, Sonko A, Faucheron JL et al. Prevalence of anal incontinence in adults and impact on quality-of-life. Gastroenterol Clin Biol. 2006; 30(1):37-43

[25] Bano F, Barrington JW. Prevalence of anorectal dysfunction in women attending health care services. Int Urogynecol J Pelvic floor Dysfunct. 2007; 18(1): 57-60.

[26] Halland M, Koloski NA, Jones M, Byles J, Chiarelli P, Forder P, Talley NJ. Prevalence correlates and impact of fecal incontinence among older women. Dis Colon Rectum. 2013 ; 56(9):1080-6.

[27] Kalantar JS, Howell S, Talley NJ. Prevalence of faecal incontinence and associated risk factors. Medical Journal of Austrália.2002; 176 (2):54-7.

[28] Lunniss PJ, Gladman MA, Franc H, Hetzer MD, Williams NS, Scott SM. Risk factors in acquired faecal incontinence. J R Soc Med. 2004; 97(3):111-6.

[29] Curti LA. Causas más frecuentes de incontinencia fecal en nuestro medio. Acta gastroenterol. Latinoam. 2000; 30(3): 165-8.

[30] Andromanakos N, Filippou D, Skandalakis P, Papadopoulos V, Rizos S, Simopoulos K. Anorectal incontinence. Pathogenesis and Choice of Treatment. J Gastrointest Liver Dis. 2006;15 (1):41-9.

[31] Fenner DE. Anal Incontinence: relationship to pregnancy, vaginal delivery, and cesarean section. Semin Perinatl. 2006 ; 30(5):261-6.

[32] Tavares DMS, Rodrigues FR, Silva CGC, Miranzi SSC. Caracterização de idosos diabéticos atendidos na atenção secundária. Ciência & Saúde Coletiva. 2007; 12(5): 1341-1352.

[33] Russo A, Botten R, Kong MF, Chapman IM, Fraser RJ, Horowitz M, et al. Effects of acute hyperglycaemia on anorectal motor and sensory function in diabetes mellitus. DiabetesMed. 2004;21(2):176-82

[34] Tieppo J, Kretzmann Filho NA, Seleme M, Fillmann HS, Berghmans B, Possa Marroni N. Anal pressure in experimental diabetes. International Journal of Colorectal Disease. 2009; 24(12): 1395-1399.

[35] Norton C, Chelvanayagam S. Conservative Management of Faecal Incontinence in adults. In: Norton C, Chelvanayagam S.Bowel Continence Nursing. UK: Beaconsfield Publishers LTD; 2004. P.114 - 131.

[36] Harari D. Bowel Care in Old Age. In: Christine Norton and Sonya Chelvanayagam. Bowel Continence Nursing. UK: Beaconsfield Publishers LTD; 2004. P.132 - 149.

[37] Bharucha AE, Fletcher Jl, Melton LJ, Zinsmeister AR. Pelvic Floor Injury and Dysfunctions in Fecal Incontinence (FI): A Population-Based Case-Control Study. Am J Gastroenterol. 2010; 138 (5): S-30.

[38] Resnick NM. Diagnosis and treatment of incontinence in the institutionalized elderly. Semin Urol. 1989;7(2):117-123.

[39] Fraga J, Azpiroz F, Malagelada J. The role of pelvic floor muscles in fecal incontinence. Gastroenterol. 2000; 118(4):126-A126

[40] Hay-Smith J, Herbison P, Morkved S. Physical therapies for prevention of urinary and faecal incontinence in adults. Cochrane Database Syst Rev. 2002(2):CD003191.

[41] Abrams P, Cardozo L, Fall M, Griffiths D, Rosier P, Ulmsten U, et al. The standardisation of terminology in lower urinary tract function: report from the standardisation sub-committee of the International Continence Society. Urology. 2003; 61(1):37-49.

[42] Schwandner O. Significance of conservative treatment for faecal incontinence. Zentralbl Chir. 2012; 137(4):323-7.

[43] Chiarioni G, Scattolini C, Bonfante F, Vantini I. Liquid stool incontinence with severe urgency: anorectal function and effective biofeedback treatment. Gut. 1993; 34(11): 1576-80.

[44] Enck P, Daublin G, Lubke HJ, Strohmeyer G. Long-term efficacy of biofeedback training for fecal incontinence. Dis Colon Rectum. 1994; 37(10):997-1001.

[45] Miner PB, Donnelly TC and Read NW. Investigation of the mode of action of biofeedback in the treatment of faecal incontinence. Digestive Diseases and Sciences. 1990; 35: 1291-8.

[46] Kegel AH. Progressive resistance exercise in the functional restoration of the perineal muscles. Am J Obst Gynecol. 1948; 56(2):238-48.

[47] Dougherty MC. Current status of research on pelvic muscle strengthening techniques. J Wound Ostomy Continence Nurs. 1998; 25(2):75-83.

[48] Miller J. Criteria for Therapeutic use of pelvic floor muscle training in women. J Wound Ostomy Continence Nurs. 2002; 29(6):301-11.

[49] Palmer MH. Pelvic muscle rehabilitation: Where do we go from here. J Wound Ostomy Cont Nurs. 1997; 24: 98-105.

[50] Griffin C, Dougherty MC, Yarandi H. Pelvic muscles during rest: responses to pelvic muscle exercise. Nurs Res. 1994; 43(3):164-7.

[51] Engel BT, Nikoomanesh P, Schuster MM. Operant conditioning of rectosphincteric responses in the treatment of fecal incontinence. N Engl J Med. 1974; 290(12):646-9.

[52] Wells TJ. Pelvic (floor) muscle exercise. J Am Geriatr Soc. 1990; 38(3):333-7.

[53] Newman DK, Fader M, Bliss DZ. Managing incontinence using technology, devices and products. Nurs Res. 2004; 53(6 suppl):S42–S48

[54] Miller J, kasper C, Sampselle C. Review of muscle physiology with application to pelvic muscle exercice. Urol Nurs. 1994; 14:92-7.

[55] Continence Foundation. Pelvic floor exercises. London: Continence Foundation; 2000.

[56] Solomon MJ, Pager CK, Rex J, Roberts R, Manning J. Randomized, controlled trial of biofeedback with anal manometry, transanal ultrasound, or pelvic floor retraining with digital guidance alone in the treatment of mild to moderate fecal incontinence. Dis Colon Rectum. 2003; 46:703–10.

[57] Norton C, Chelvanayagam S. Methodology of Biofeedback for Fecal Adults With Fecal Incontinence: A Program of Care. Journal of Wound, ostomy and Continence Nursing. 2001; 28(3):156-68.

[58] Norton C, Whitehe WE, Bliss DZ, Harari D, Lang J. Management of Fecal in adults. Neurol Urodynamics. 2010;29:199-206.

[59] Doughty DB, Burns P. Pathology and Management of Stress Incontinence. In: Doughty DB, editor: Urinary and fecal incontinence: nursing management, 2nd ed, St. Louis: Mosby; 2000. p. 77-107.

[60] Evans G. Pelvic-floor exercises for incontinence. Women's Health Medicine. 2005; 2(6):29-30.

[61] Norton C, Christiansen J, Butler U, Harari D, Nelson R, Pemberton JH, Price K, Rovner ES, Sultan AH. Anal incontinence. In: Abrams P, Khoury S, Wein A, Cardozo L, Editors, Incontinence, Plymouth: Health Books; 2002.

[62] Tan JJY, Chan M, Tjandra JJ. Evolving Therapy for Fecal Incontinence. Dis Colon Rectum. 2007; 50(11):1264-72.

[63] Sobrado CW, Miszputenm SJ. Constipação intestinal. In: Amaro JL. et al. Reabilitação do assoalho pélvico nas funções urinárias e anorretais. São Paulo: Segmento Farma. 2005. p. 285-309.

[64] Chiarioni G, Ferri B, Morelli A, Iantorno G, Bassotti G. Bio-feedback treatment of fecal incontinence: where are we, and where are we going? World J Gastroenterol. 2005; 11(31):4771-5.

[65] Whitehead WE, Drossman DA. Biofeedback for disorders of elimination: Fecal incontinence and pelvic floor dyssynergia. Profes Psychol: Research and Practice. 1996;27(3):234-40.

[66] Lima TGS, Santos VLCG, Lacombe DLP, Manso JEF. Incontinência Anal: Tratamento conservador por meio de Biofeedback. Rev Estima. 2010; 8(3):42-4.

[67] Netinho JG, Dourado HM, Starling F, Ramalho EN. Tratamento da Incontinência Anal com Biofeedback: Resultados preliminares. Ver Bras Coloproct. 1999; 19(2): 89-93.

[68] Ozturk R, Niazi S, Stessman M, Rao SSC. Long-term outcome and objective changes of anorectal function after biofeedback therapy for faecal incontinence. Aliment Pharmacol Ther. 2004; 20:667–74.

[69] Chiarioni G, Bassotti G, Stanganini S, Vantini I, Whitehead WE. Sensory retraining is key to biofeedback therapy for formed stool fecal incontinence. Am J Gastroenterol. 2002;97(1):109-17.

[70] Dobben AC, Terra MP, Berghmans B, Deutekom M, Boeckxstaens GE, Janssen LW, et al. Functional changes after physiotherapy in fecal incontinence. Int J Colorectal Dis. 2006; 21(6):515-21

[71] Byrne CM, Solomon MJ, Rex J, Young JM, Heggie D, Merlino C. Telephone vs. face-to-face biofeedback for fecal incontinence: comparison of two techniques in 239 patients. Dis Colon Rectum. 2005; 48(12):2281-8.

[72] Martínez-Puente MC, Pascual-Montero JA, García-Olmo D. Customized biofeedback therapy improves results in fecal incontinence. Int J Colorectal Dis. 2004; 19:210-14

[73] Bartlett L, Nowak M, Ho YH. Impact of fecal incontinence on quality of life. World J Gastroenterol. 2009; 15(26):3276-82.

[74] Lima TGS, Santos VLCG, Lacombe DLP, Manso JEF. Eficácia do Biofeedback por orientação digital e manométrico em pacientes com incontinência anal. Tese de Doutorado. 2011.

[75] Mergulhão MEA. Eletroestimulação, biofeedback e associação de eletroestimulação com biofeedback no tratamento da incontinência fecal [Dissertação]. Campinas: Faculdade de Ciências Médicas, Universidade Estadual de Campinas; 2004.

[76] Norton C, Whitehead W, Bliss DZ, Harari D Lang J. Conservative and Pharmacological Management of Faecal Incontinence in Adults. In: Abrams P, Cardozo L, Khoury S, Wein A, eds. Incontinence. Plymouth: Health Publications, 2009: 1323–86. [cited 2013 Sep. 04]. Avalilable from: http://www.ics.org/Publications/ICI_4/book.pdf

[77] Norton C, Gibbs A, Kamm MA Randomized, Controlled Trial of Anal Electrical Stimulation for Fecal Incontinence. Diseases of the Colon & Rectum. 2006;49(2):190-6.

[78] Brito CMM, Schmidt FMQ, Canettieri MG, de La Quintana MM, Andrade PAS, Gimenez TM. Reabilitação da Disfunção Vesicoesfincteriana. In: Brito CMM, Bazan M, Pinto C, Baia W, Battistella LR. Manual de Reabilitação em Oncologia do Instituto do Câncer do Estado de São Paulo (ICESP). São Paulo: Manole; 2013. In press.

[79] Mahony RT, Malone PA, Nalty J, Behan M, O'Connell PR, O'Herlihy C. Randomized clinical trial of intra-anal electromyographic biofeedback physiotherapy with intra-anal electromyographic biofeedback augmented with electrical stimulation of the anal sphincter in the early treatment of postpartum fecal incontinence. American Journal of Obstetrics and Gynecology. 2004; 191:885-90.

[80] Hosker G, Cody JD, Norton CC. Electrical stimulation for faecal incontinence in adults. Cochrane Database of Systematic Reviews 2007, Issue 3. Art. No.: CD001310. DOI: 0.1002/14651858.CD001310.pub2.

[81] Costilla C, Foxx-orenstein E, Mayer P, Crowell M. office-based management of fecal incontinence. Gastroenterol Hepatol. 2013 jul;9(7):423-33.

[82] Kenefick NJ. Sacral Nerve Neuromodulation for the Treatment of Lower Bowel Motility Disorders. Ann R Coll Surg Engl. 2006;88(7): 617–623.

[83] Mowatt G, Glazener CMA, Jarrett M. Sacral nerve stimulation for faecal incontinence and constipation in adults. Cochrane Database of Systematic Reviews 2007, Issue 3. Art. No.: CD004464. DOI: 10.1002/14651858.CD004464.pub2

[84] Ratto C, Parello A, Donisi L, Doglietto GB. Sacral neuromodulation in the treatment of defecation disorders. Acta Neurochir Suppl. 2007;97(Pt 1):341-50.

[85] Schreiner L. Eletroestimulação do nervo tibial no tratamento da incontinência urinária de urgência em idosas [Dissertação]. Porto Alegre: Pontifícia Universidade Católica do Rio Grande do Sul; 2009.

[86] Souza GP, Suter TMC, Tonon E. Tratamento fisioterapêutico em incontinência fecal com estimulação elétrica do nervo tibial posterior e cinesioterapia: relato de caso. Revista Hórus. 2011;5(3). [cited 2013 Sep. 04]. Avalilable from: http://www.faeso.edu.br/horus/artigos%20anteriores/2011/CAP5.pdf

Chapter 8

Anal Injectables and Implantables for Faecal Incontinence

John Camilleri-Brennan

Additional information is available at the end of the chapter

http://dx.doi.org/10.5772/58327

1. Introduction

Faecal Incontinence (FI) can have an adverse effect on quality of life. It is a stigmatising condition that may lead to severe social restriction. From the financial point of view, the investigation and treatment of faecal incontinence may add to a significant cost to the health systems of most countries. In fact, the annual treatment cost of patients in the U.K. with urinary and faecal incontinence is of about £500 million.

Many factors may be involved in the pathophysiology of FI. A thorough clinical assessment of the patient is therefore mandatory. This starts with a full history, which may include a cognitive assessment if necessary. The characteristics of the faeces and the type and frequency of incontinence should be noted. Urge incontinence is suggestive of poor external anal sphincter function, whilst passive and post-defaecatory incontinence indicate that internal anal sphincter function is weak. Various questionnaires that enable the clinician to quantify the degree of incontinence and the impact on quality of life are available. These include symptom-specific questionnaires, such as the ones developed by Vaizey et al [1] and Wexner et al [2], the Faecal Incontinence Quality of Life Scale (FIQOL) developed by Rockwood et al [3], and also generic questionnaires such as the Short Form 36 (SF 36) [4].

A full examination of the patient, including the abdomen and perineum, and a neurological examination in some cases, is necessary. Beneficial investigations include a flexible sigmoidoscopy, anal manometry (resting and squeeze pressure), rectal compliance, pudendal nerve terminal motor latency (PNTML) and endoanal ultrasound.

The management of FI is usually multidisciplinary, involving the general practitioner, continence nurse, physiotherapist, gastroenterologist, urologist and colorectal surgeon.

Conservative measures, which include patient education and support, improvement in diet and bowel habit, judicious use of anti-diarrhoeal medication and pelvic floor exercises, are used in the first instance. This is, in fact, recommended in the UK by the National Institute for Clinical Excellence (NICE) guideline 'CG49 Faecal Incontinence' [5]. If these measures fail, however, surgical intervention may be necessary. A variety of surgical options are available, with the appropriate therapy being selected depending on the cause of the incontinence and the patient's cognitive function and general physical condition (Table 1). One of the surgical options available is the use of anal bulking agents.

1. Restoration and improvement of residual sphincter function
a. Correcting a defective External Anal Sphincter: Sphincteroplasty (End-to-end repair; Overlap repair)
b. Correcting a defective Pelvic Floor:
Levatorplasty
Postanal Repair
Total Pelvic Floor Repair
c. Correction of Anorectal Deformities
d. Sacral Nerve Stimulation (SNS)
e. Posterior Tibial Nerve Stimulation (PTNS)
2. Increasing the outlet resistance of the anal sphincter
a. Augmentation of the Anal Sphincter and Anal Cushions (Anal Bulking Agents)
b. Anal Submucosal Fibrosis (SECCA)
c. Anal Encirclement (Thiersch procedure)
d. Non-Dynamic Graciloplasty
3. Dynamic Sphincter Replacement
a. Dynamic Graciloplasty
b. Artificial Anal Sphincter
4. Antegrade Continence Enema (ACE)
5. Faecal Diversion
a. Colostomy
b. Ileostomy

Table 1. Surgical Options in the Management of Faecal Incontinence

http://dx.doi.org/10.5772/58327

2. Anal bulking agents

Anal bulking agents have emerged as a treatment for F.I. following the success of bulking agents for urinary stress incontinence in females. In the urology setting, bulking agents have been employed to augment the bladder neck and increase urethral resistance [6]. Therefore, the aim of anal bulking agents is to prevent F.I. by closing the anal canal or increasing the pressure within the anal sphincter.

The ideal characteristics of a bulking agent have been described in the literature [7]. The injected or implanted substance should be biocompatible, non-migratory, non-allergenic and non-carcinogenic. The substance should also be easy to inject or implant and should produce an improvement in continence, both in the short-term as well as in the long-term.

The evidence for anal bulking agents

Anal injectables and implantables have been used to manage faecal incontinence for over 20 years. It may be useful to chart their development over the years and to classify this development into three phases. The first phase consists of the initial experimental studies that took place in the nineties. The second phase, from about the year 2000 onwards, encompasses an increase in the number of studies using a wide variety of agents and injection techniques. The third phase features the latest generation of anal bulking agents, the implantable THD Gatekeeper.

2.1. Initial studies: The first phase

Anal bulking agents were first described in 1993 by Shafik [8]. Shafik, an Egyptian surgeon, is considered to be a pioneer in this field. In his first study, he described the outcomes following the injection of 5ml of PTFE (Polytef / Teflon) paste in 11 patients, 7 of whom had incontinence following a lateral internal sphincterotomy for anal fissure. In another study, the same author used 60 ml of abdominal wall fat as a submucosal injection into the rectal neck at 3 and 9 o'clock in 14 patients with partial faecal incontinence [9]. Pescatori's group from Rome, Italy, reported the use of anal injection of autologous buttock fat to restore continence in one patient who had poor results following a sphincteroplasty. This patient's continence improved following repeated injections [10].

The indications for injection of the anal bulking agents in these studies were various. Most patients had passive FI, but some had urge incontinence, indicating EAS disruption. The results of these initial studies showed that continence was improved in the short term. However, the medium and long-term results were poor, probably because of resorbtion or migration of the injected material. Re-injection was necessary in order to maintain continence.

A number of safety issues were raised with these studies. Teflon could potentially cause granuloma formation and sarcomas. The injection of autologous fat as a bulking agent in urology has been implicated in fatal fat embolism and stroke.

2.2. The second phase

The second phase in the development of anal bulking agents consisted of a wide variation in the types of materials used, surgical technique and clinical indications [11]. Some of the materials used to bulk the anal sphincter were being used in urology to augment the bladder neck. Nine different types of injectable bulking agents have been used in these studies (Table 2).

Type of Bulking agent	Commercial name/s	Injection site	Injection route	Published studies	No. of patients
Silicone biomaterial. Polydimethylsiloxane elastomer particles suspended in a biocompatible hydrogel made of poly-N-vinyl-pyrrolidone	PTQ; Bioplastique	Intersphincteric ; within IAS	Transsphincteric	21	619
Carbon-coated zirconium beads, comprised of pyrolytic carbon-coated beads suspended in a water-based carrier gel containing β-glucan	Durasphere	Submucosal	Transmucosal; Transsphincteric	7	187
Spherical particles of calcium hydroxylapatite, suspended in a gel carrier	Coaptite	Submucosal	Transsphincteric	1	10
Dextranomer microspheres and stabilized sodium hyaluronate in phosphate-buffered 0.9% sodium chloride solution	NASHA Dx, Zuidex, Solesta	Submucosal	Transmucosal	4	56
Glutaraldehyde cross-linked collagen	Contigen	Submucosal	Transmucosal	2	90
Synthetic non-particulate hydrogel consisting of water (97.5%) and cross-linked polyacrylamide (2·5%)	Bulkamid	Intersphincteric	Intersphincteric	1	5
Cross-linked porcine dermal collagen matrix	Permacol	Submucosal; Intersphincteric	Transmucosal; Intersphincteric	5	172
8% Ethylene Vinyl alcohol co-polymer dissolved in dimethyl sulphoxide. A spongy solid mass forms from the solidification of the hydrophobic co-polymer when the solvent diffuses away on contact with tissue fluid	Onyx34	Intershincteric	Intersphincteric	1	21
Expandable silicone Microballoons filled with a biocompatible hydrogel made of poly-N-vinyl-pyrrolidone		Submucosal	Transmucosal	1	6

Table 2. Injectable materials used in the second phase of studies

http://dx.doi.org/10.5772/58327

Indications:

The clinical indications for which these bulking agents were used varied from study to study. These were:

- Failure of conservative management of faecal incontinence
- Structurally intact but weak internal anal sphincter (IAS). This would be due to either primary idiopathic degeneration of the IAS, or degeneration secondary to tissue disorders such as scleroderma
- IAS damage (childbirth, haemorrhoidectomy, anal stretch, sphincterotomy) (Figure 1)
- Defect in the external anal sphincter (EAS)

The main indication was IAS dysfunction or disruption. Unlike the EAS, the IAS is not amenable to surgical repair.

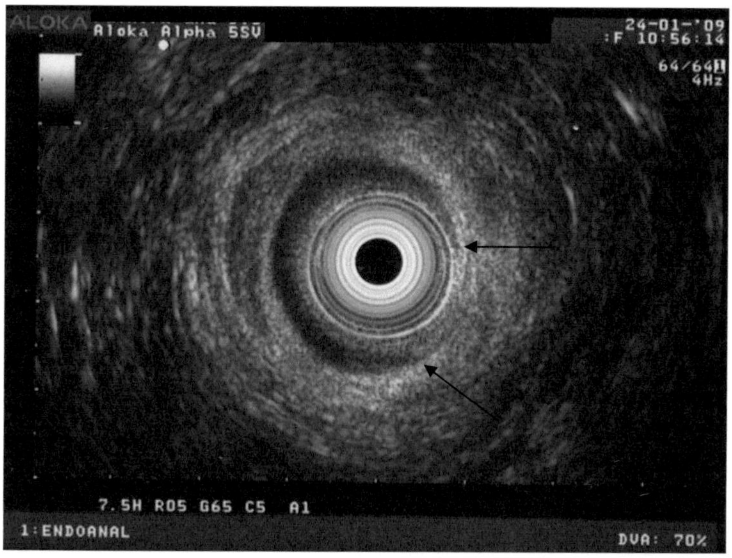

Figure 1. Endoanal ultrasound scan showing a defect in the IAS of a 57year old lady with passive faecal incontinence following haemorrhoidectomy. The defect is present between the arrows from the 3 to the 5 o'clock positions.

Surgical Procedure and Technique:

The bulking agents may be inserted under local, regional (anal or pudendal nerve block) or general anaesthesia. The type of anaesthesia used depends on the preference of the patient and the surgeon. The patient may be positioned in the prone (jack-knife), lithothomy or left lateral positions, although the latter position may not give a satisfactory view of the anorectum to enable accurate injection. A phosphate enema is usually administered preoperatively. The procedure is usually covered by prophylactic antibiotics, such as intravenous (IV) Co-amoxiclav 1.2g, Cefuroxime 750mg and Metronidazole 500mg or Gentamicin 1.5mg/kg and Metronidazole 500mg at induction.

The injection of the bulking agent varies depending on the type of substance used and the clinical indications. Three different routes of needle insertion were mentioned in the literature: transmucosal, trans-sphincteric or intersphincteric. The bulking agent was placed submucosally, within the intersphincteric space or within the IAS itself. For example, porcine dermal collagen (Permacol) may be injected via the transmucosal or trans-sphincteric route using a disposable 19G needle [12] (Figure 2). In patients with an intact IAS, 2.5ml of Permacol is equally injected into the submucosal space at the 3, 7 and 11 o'clock positions above the dentate line. In cases of an IAS defect, 5ml of Permacol may be injected at the site of the defect, with 2.5ml of the substance injected diametrically opposite. With silicone biomaterial (PTQ or Bioplastique), four doses of 2.5ml of silicone are used, using an 18G needle [13, 14]. Patients with an intact IAS have the silicone injected trans-sphincterically into the intersphincteric space at the 2, 4, 8 and 10 o'clock positions. In patients with an IAS defect, for example after a lateral internal sphincterotomy, a total of three doses of 2.5 ml of silicone are injected into the defect. A fourth dose is injected into the intersphincteric space contralateral to the IAS defect, to provide symmetry. With carbon-coated beads (Durasphere) a total of 10ml are injected in four divided doses in the submucosal plane using an 18G needle [14].

It is of utmost importance to ensure that the anal mucosa is not breached during injection, since that would allow intra-anal leakage of the substance. Intravascular injection must also be avoided.

Once the injection is completed, it is good practice to leave the needle and syringe in place for a few seconds. As the needle is being withdrawn, pressure on the needle track by the index finger may prevent leakage of the bulking agent [12].

The bulking agent may be injected freehand, with an anal retractor such as Eisenhammer used to identify the IAS and intersphincteric groove. A finger placed within the anal canal may be useful to guide the needle to its correct position. However endoanal ultrasound has been recommended to guide the needle to an optimum position [13], especially if the agent is to be injected into the intersphincteric space or adjacent to a defect in the IAS.

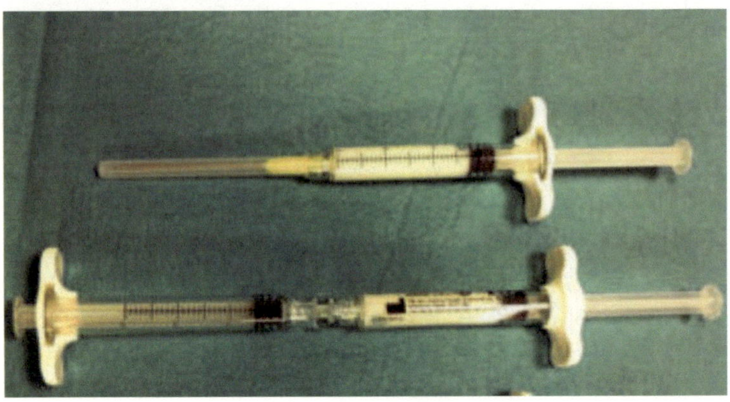

Figure 2. Porcine dermal collagen (Permacol) in a 2.5ml syringe

http://dx.doi.org/10.5772/58327

Results:

The majority of studies in this second phase of development were mainly case series and observational studies. Most of these studies reported either an improvement in the faecal continence scores or less frequent episodes of incontinence over time. Anorectal manometry testing featured in some studies, with some showing an improvement in resting or squeeze pressures. Others studies showed no such improvement. Clinical improvement was not always associated with an increase in these pressures. Quality of life was formally assessed in some of these studies. The majority reported an improvement across various domains such as physical and social function.

To date there have been five randomised trials using anal bulking agents, with a total of 382 patients. Two trials compared a bulking agent with a sham or saline injection. Siproudhis et al in 2007 [15] compared a silicone biomaterial (PTQ) with a normal saline injection (control) into the intersphincteric space. PTQ did not demonstrate any appreciable clinical benefit when compared to the control. The trial was however deemed to be too small to detect any differences in continence. Graf et al in 2011[16] compared the injection of dextranomer (NASHADx) against sham injection (no substance injected). Continence was better in the short term (6 months) in the active intervention group, although interestingly about 30% of patients in the control group had an improvement in their continence.

A small study with ten patients by Maeda et al in 2008 [17] revealed significant improvement at 6 weeks post injection using injection of Bulkamid and Permacol. Continence decreased slightly in the Permacol group at 6 months. However there was no reported difference between the two agents. The numbers were too small to detect a difference. Tjandra et al in 2009, reported the results of a randomised study comparing PTQ with carbon-coated beads (Durasphere) [14]. PTQ injection was associated with better continence scores and quality of life, and was safer, than Durasphere.

Tjandra et al in 2004 reported the short-term benefits from ultrasound guided injection of silicone biomaterial (PTQ) compared with digital guidance [13].

The follow up for the majority of patients in studies was less than a median of 3 years. A question on the term durability and effectiveness of these agents is therefore raised. The majority (97%) of patients were only followed up once or twice. No long-term evidence on outcomes was available and further conclusions were not warranted from the available data. None of the studies reported patient evaluation of outcomes and thus it is difficult to gauge whether the improvement in the continence scores matched the practical symptom and quality of life improvements that mattered to the patients.

The majority of patients did not report any complications. The complications described were mainly pain, anal bruising and leakage of injected material [11, 12]. Less common complications were anal ulceration and infection (local cellulitis and abscess formation). There were two reported cases of local giant cell foreign body reaction after injection of silicone (PTQ)[18]. Durasphere has been associated with skin rashes and arthritis. Skin patch testing is therefore recommended before using this agent [14].

2.3. The third phase: The implantable THD Gatekeeper

A relatively new and innovative development in anal bulking technology is the THD Gatekeeper (THD S.p.A., Correggio, Italy). The material used is Polyacrylonitrile or Hyexpan. It is an inert, non-allergenic, non-degradable material that is also non-immunogenic, and non-carcinogenic. First developed by Medtronic in Minneapolis, USA, it was originally used as an implant in the oesophagogastric junction for the management of gastro-oesophageal reflux disease.

The main indications for the use of the THD Gatekeeper are passive faecal incontinence, secondary to IAS dysfunction or damage, where conservative measures or injection of other bulking agents such as PTQ or Permacol have failed.

The following are contraindications to the use of the Gatekeeper. Similar contraindications have also been described by the product manufacturers of other anal bulking agents.

- Perianal sepsis
- Inflammatory bowel diseases with anorectal involvement (Crohn's disease, ulcerative colitis)
- Anal cancer
- Rectal or colon cancer undergoing active treatment;
- Rectal bleeding of unknown or undiagnosed origin;
- Rectal prolapse
- Uncontrolled blood coagulation disorders
- Pelvic radiotherapy
- Immunosuppression
- Pregnancy or planned pregnancy in the next 12 months.

Surgical Apparatus, Procedure and Technique:

Whereas the anal bulking agents that were developed in phases 1 and 2 are injected into or around the anal canal by means of a hypodermic syringe, the Hyexpan prostheses are implanted into the intersphincteric space using a custom-made gun (Figure 3).

The prostheses consist of thin solid cylinders, 22mm long and 2mm in diameter. The success of this material depends on its hydrophilic properties. Within 24 hours after implantation in human tissue, the Hyexpan cylinders absorb water to become thicker and shorter. The *in vitro* maximum diameter is 6.5 mm and the length is 17 mm (Figure 4). The volume of each individual implant increases from approximately 70mm^3 to 500mm^3, a 750% increase. The implant is also much softer in consistency compared to the firm consistency prior to implantation.

http://dx.doi.org/10.5772/58327

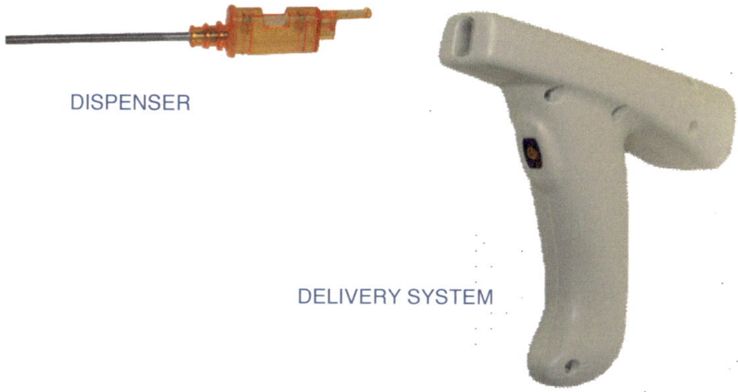

Figure 3. The Gatekeeper gun, made of the dispenser that houses one prosthesis, and the delivery system.

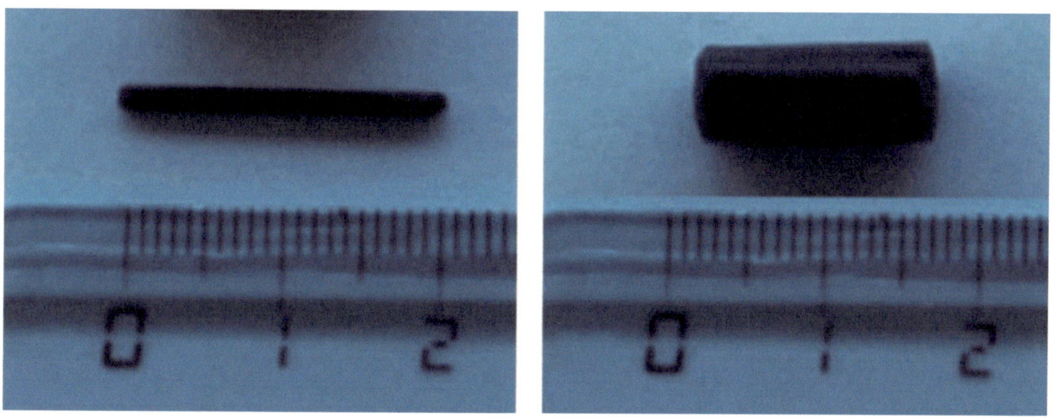

Figure 4. a. Shape of Hyexpan cylinders at insertion. b. Fully expanded Hyexpan cylinder following contact with water

The operation is performed under regional or general anesthesia. Intravenous antibiotics are given at induction. The author's patients receive Gentamicin 1.5 mg/kg and Metronidazole 500mg IV. The patient is placed in the lithotomy position. A strict sterile technique is used. The IAS and intersphincteric groove are identified by the placement of an anal retractor (eg. Eisenhammer or Park's). The author's preference is a THD surgy Mini-light proctoscope, a self illuminating anal and rectal retractor that gives a very good view of the anorectum without causing trauma to the anal sphincter (Figure 5).

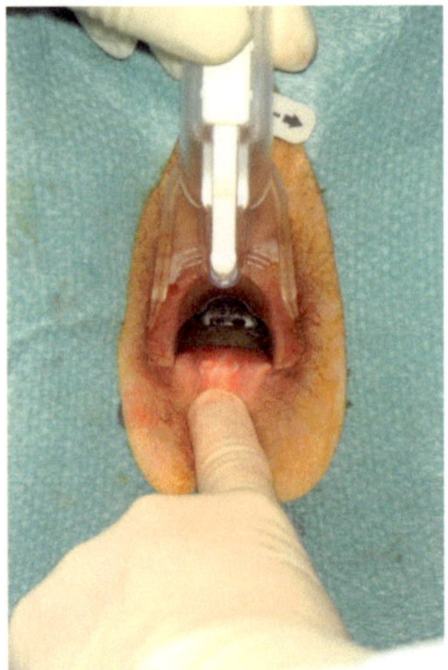

Figure 5. Palpating the IAS and the intersphincteric groove at the 6 o'clock position with a THD surgy Mini-light proctoscope in position.

A 2mm incision is made in the perianal skin, 2 cm from the anal verge (Figure 6).

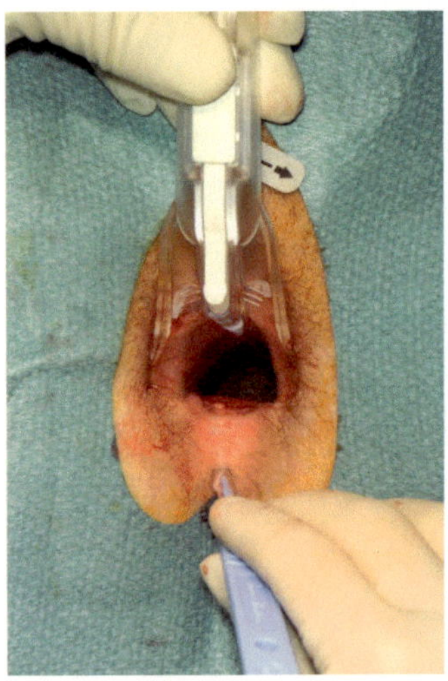

Figure 6. Making an incision, 2cm away from the anal verge, at the 6 o'clock position.

Having attached the dispenser to the delivery system, the needle is inserted through the incision and tunneled to the intersphincteric margin and introduced into the intersphincteric space. The needle is then positioned so that the tip would lie just beyond the dentate line. When the needle is identified in the correct position, by direct vision and palpation and/or by endoanal ultrasound, the prosthesis is released into the intersphincteric space (Figure 7).

http://dx.doi.org/10.5772/58327

The steps may be repeated to insert between four to six prostheses, equidistant from each other. The choice of inserting 4 as opposed to 6 prostheses is arbitrary. The wounds are closed with a single absorbable suture (Figure 8). At the end of procedure, EAUS imaging will show the location of all prostheses.

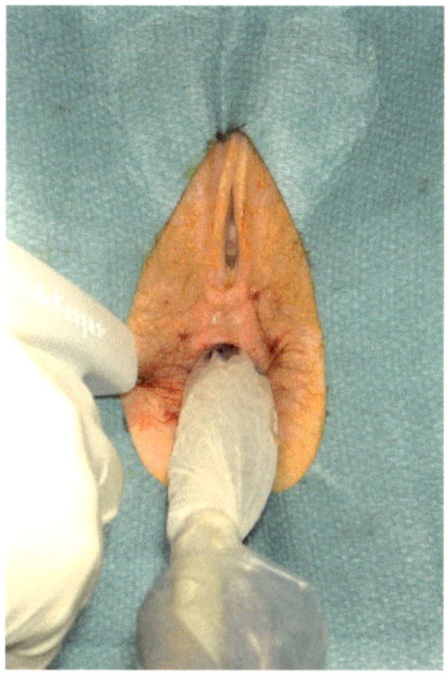

Figure 7. THD Gatekeeper needle at the 9 o'clock position, with the endoanal ultrasound probe in place to determine correct placement.

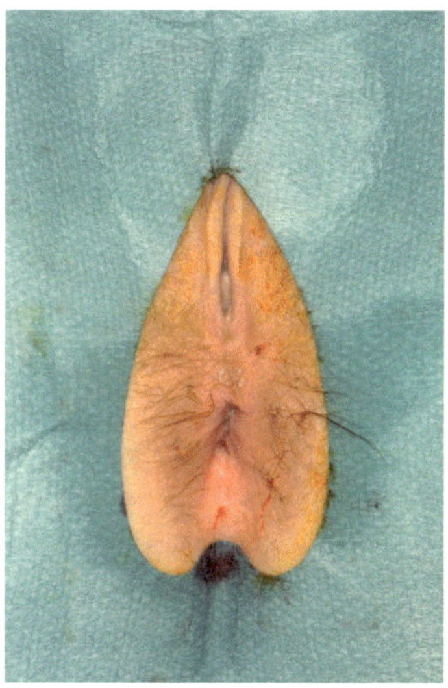

Figure 8. Six equidistant circumferential perianal wounds each closed with an absorbable suture (Monocryl 3/0).

The procedure takes about 30 to 40 minutes to complete, and is done as a day-case. Oral metronidazole 400mg tds is prescribed for 5 days postoperatively. Oral laxatives such as lactulose are prescribed to minimize the risk of constipation. The patients are advised to avoid any anal trauma as well as anal intercourse for at least 72 h after implant insertion.

The patients are followed up after 6 weeks and 3 monthly thereafter.

The material remains identifiable both by palpation and by endoanal ultrasonography in the postoperative period (Figure 9).

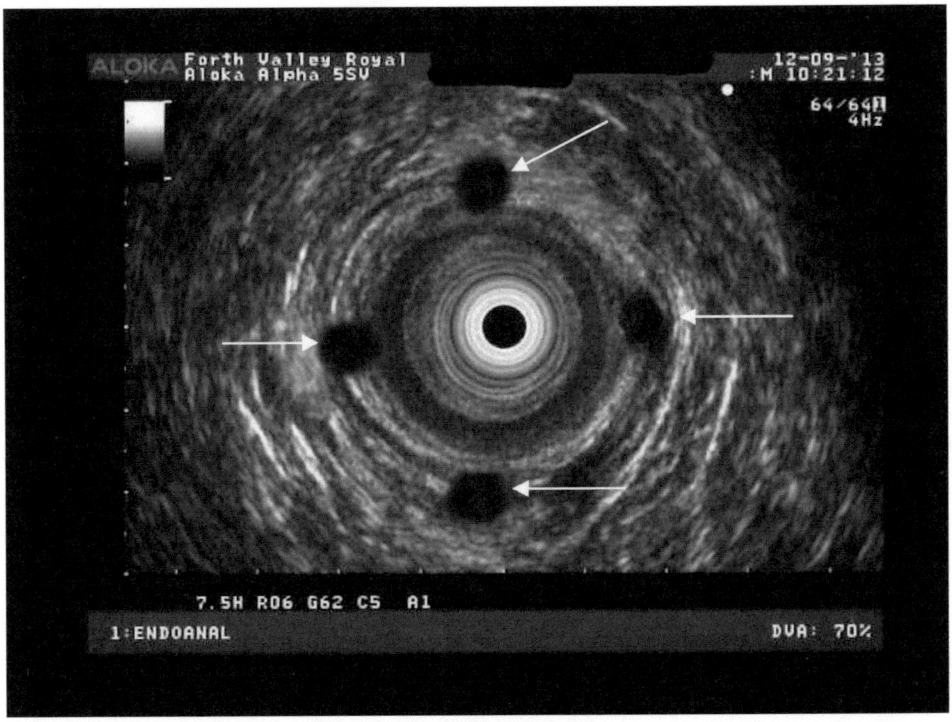

Figure 9. Endoanal ultrasound scan at 6 weeks following the implantation of four Gatekeeper prostheses (arrows) in a 72 year old male with idiopathic passive faecal incontinence.

Results:

The first reported experience with the THD Gatekeeper was by Ratto et al in 2011 [19]. This was a study with 14 patients. Eight had idiopathic FI, 4 had an IAS defect and 2 had combined IAS and EAS defects. The median follow-up was of 12 months (range 5 to 48 months). The authors reported a clinically significant improvement in continence in 13 patients, a sustained significant improvement in the Wexner and Vaizey scores and in the SF36 and FIQL quality of life scores. No complications have been reported.

The second study was a comparative retrospective study by Parello et al in 2012 [20]. Seven patients who had the THD Gatekeeper implanted were compared to 6 patients who underwent sacral nerve stimulation (SNS). The median follow up was of 18 months in the Gatekeeper group and 20 months in the SNS group. The authors reported a sustained improvement in the Wexner continence scores with both modalities of treatment.

The results of the author's first 5 patients using this novel technique were evaluated. One was male and 4 were female. Four had idiopathic FI and one had passive incontinence following anal strech for anal fissure. All patients had failed conservative management. There was a significant impovement in median Vaizey scores at 6 months (16 vs 4, $p<0.01$). One patient, who was assessed at 12 months, had a sustained score improvement from 14 at baseline to 3 at 3, 6 and 12 months. There have not been any complications to date.

3. Discussion

The development of anal injectable and implantable technology over the past 20 years has taken great strides forwards. Starting with the pioneering efforts of Shafik with autologous fat, more materials have been tried and used, the more popular being Collagen (Permacol) and Silicone (PTQ or Bioplastique). These agents were associated with variable and inconsistent results. Injections were frequently repeated to maintain continence long term. The latest generation of anal bulking agents is the implantable Hyexpan (THD Gatekeeper). This material fits the criteria for the 'ideal' bulking agent. It overcomes most limitations of other bulking agents, and its use has shown very promising initial results. Whether these results are maintained in the longer term or not awaits to be seen.

The mechanism of action of anal bulking agents is a subject of debate. Most of the resting anal pressure is the function of the IAS, with some contribution from the EAS and anal cushions. Studies of faecal incontinence in patients who have undergone a traditional Milligan Morgan haemorrhoidectomy lend support the concept that anal cushions play an important part in the maintenance of the normal mechanism of continence. It is thought that the mechanism of action of a bulking agent injected into the submucosal space is an increase in the size of the natural anal cushions. On the other hand, a bulking agent injected or implanted into the intersphincteric space would bulk the size of the anal sphincter. The end result would be an improvement in the seal of the lumen of the anal canal at rest and potentially an increase in resting anal pressure and in the length of the anal high pressure zone. When the injection is placed adjacent to an identifiable IAS defect, a better degree of anal canal sealing may be obtained through improvement in the configuration and symmetry of the anal canal [7].

It is acknowledged that more research required in this field. Most studies are case series with very few randomised trials.

Larger series with longer follow up and randomised controlled trials are therefore necessary. Further development on existing and emerging technology is also warranted.

Author details

John Camilleri-Brennan[1,2*]

Address all correspondence to: johncbrennan@doctors.org.uk

1 Department of Surgery, Forth Valley Royal Hospital, Larbert, Stirlingshire, Scotland

2 University of Glasgow Medical School, Glasgow, Scotland

References

[1] Vaizey CJ, Carapeti E, Cahill JA, and Kamm MA. Prospective comparison of faecal incontinence grading systems. Gut Jan 1999; 44: 77 – 80.

[2] Jorge, J.M.N., Wexner, S.D.: Etiology and management of fecal incontinence. Dis. Colon Rectum 36:77-97, 1993.

[3] Rockwood TH, Church JM, Fleshman JW, et al. Fecal Incontinence Quality of Life Scale: quality of life instrument for patients with fecal incontinence. Dis Colon Rectum. 2000; 43(1):9-17

[4] Ware JE Jr, Sherbourne CD. The MOS 36-item short-form health survey (SF-36). I. Conceptual framework and item selection. Med Care 1992; 30:473–83

[5] National Institute for Clinical Excellence (NICE). The management of faecal incontinence in adults. Clinical Guideline 49 NICE 2007

[6] Lightner DJ. Review of the available urethral bulking agents. Curr Opin Urol 2002.12:333–338

[7] Vaizey CJ, Kamm MA. Injectable bulking agents for treating faecal incontinence. Br J Surg 2005; 92: 521-7.

[8] Shafik A. Polytetrafluoroethylene injection for the treatment of partial fecal incontinence. Int Surg 1993; 78: 159–91.

[9] Shafik A. Perianal injection of autologous fat for treatment of sphincteric incontinence. Dis Colon Rectum 1995; 38: 583–7.

[10] Bernardi C, Favetta U, Pescatori M. Autologous fat injection for treatment of fecal incontinence: manometric and echographic essment. Plast Reconstr Surg 1998; 102: 1626–8.

[11] Maeda Y, Laurberg S, Norton C. Perianal injectable bulking agents as treatment for faecal incontinence in adults. Cochrane Database Syst Rev. 2010;(5):CD007959.

[12] Watson NFS, Koshy A and Sagar PM. Anal bulking agents for faecal incontinence. Colorectal Disease 2012. 14 (Suppl. 3), 29–33.

[13] Tjandra JJ, Lim JF, Hiscock R, Rajendra P. Injectable silicone biomaterial for fecal incontinence caused by internal l sphincter dysfunction is effective. Dis Colon Rectum 2004; 47: 2138–46.

[14] Tjandra JJ, Chan MK, Yeh HC. Injectable silicone biomaterial (PTQ) is more effective than carbon-coated beads (Durasphere) in treating passive faecal incontinence-a randomized trial. Colorectal Disease 2009;11(4):382–9.

[15] Siproudhis L, Morcet J, Laine F. Elastomer implants in faecal incontinence: a blind, randomized placebo-controlled study. Alimentary Pharmacology & Therapeutics 2007;25(9): 1125–32.

[16] Graf W, Mellgren A, Matzel KE, Hull T, Johansson C, Bernstein M, et al. Efficacy of dextranomer in stabilised hyaluronic acid for treatment of faecal incontinence: a randomised, sham-controlled trial. *Lancet* 2011;377(9770): 997–1003.

[17] Maeda Y, Vaizey CJ, Kamm MA. Pilot study of two new injectable bulking agents for the treatment of faecal incontinence. Colorectal Disease 2008; 10(3):268–72.

[18] van Wunnik B, Driessen A, Baeten C. Local giant cell foreign body reaction after silicone injection for fecal incontinence in humans: two case reports. Tech Coloproctol 2012. 16:395–397

[19] Ratto C, Parello A, Donisi L, Litta F, De Simone V, Spazzafumo L, Giordano P. Novel bulking agent for faecal incontinence. British Journal of Surgery 2011; 98 (11): 1644–52

[20] Parello A, De Simone V, Donisi L, Litta F, Zaccone, Ratto C. Can Gatekeper, a new bulking agent be equivalent to SNS in patients with fecal incontinence in the presence of only internal sphincter defects. Tech Coloproctol 2012. 16:77

Chapter 9

Traumatic Cloaca

Constantine P. Spanos

Additional information is available at the end of the chapter

http://dx.doi.org/10.5772/57377

1. Introduction

Traumatic cloacal deformities are a result of major obstetric injury; these usually occur after a fourth-degree perineal laceration. They occur in one in 5000 vaginal deliveries. [1] This deformity is characterized by three anatomic lesions: complete disruption of the perineal body, anterior defect of the internal and external anal sphincter, and loss of the distal rectovaginal and/or anovaginal septum. [2-4] Thus, a common genitourinary and gastrointestinal outlet ensues, as in congenital cloaca. This is the cause of symptoms and disorders related to this condition.

Resulting disorders are mostly functional. These patients suffer from severe incontinence to flatus, liquid and solid stool. Recurrent urinary tract and vaginal infection may also result. Sexual dysfunction is significant; patients often complain of dyspareunia [4] or refrain from sexual activity altogether. Partners are also affected. All these disorders may lead to psychological disorders and social distress associated with incapacitating incontinence as well as a sense of shame from the "deformity". [3-6] A nihilistic approach from both the patient and physicians may lead to delay in treatment, thus burdening the patient with years of suffering and diminished quality of life.

There are several reports and series in the literature describing techniques for repairing traumatic cloacal deformities. There is considerable variety regarding the use or not of flaps, the use or not of fecal diversion. In any case, repair of these deformities can be challenging and complex, and patients may present years after the initial injury. Some may have had a previous repair, thus adding difficulty to definitive correction.

2. Etiology

Traumatic cloaca is usually the result of obstetric injury. The most common injuries involved are third and fourth-degree perineal lacerations. Third-degree lacerations are characterized by disruption of the internal and external anal sphincter. In fourth-degree lacerations, disruption of the anal and/or rectal epithelium is included in addition to sphincter injury. Surgical correction of these types of injuries involves precise, layered approximation of damaged structures and tissues. Failure of repair may be a result of hematoma, infection or technical mishaps. Partial failure may result in a rectovaginal fistula; complete failure leads to a cloacal deformity. [8] Traumatic cloaca may occur if these obstetric injuries of this nature are not repaired, or after failure of surgical repair. This may be secondary to poor surgical technique or a complication such as infection and disruption of the layered repair.

The resulting deformity is three-dimensional absence of the perineal body, disruption of the sphincter complex and loss of the anovaginal/anorectal septum of varying length.

3. Signs and symptoms

Most, if not all, women with traumatic cloacae have severe incontinence to flatus, liquid and solid stool. These patients also suffer from sequelae of the communication of the gastrointestinal and genitourinary tract; namely, severe perineal skin irritation, as well as recurrent urinary tract and vaginal infections. Sexual function is seriously affected. Many patients complain of dyspareunia, and abstinence from sexual activity is not uncommon. Thus, spouses and sexual partners are also affected by this disorder.

Traumatic cloaca may lead to psychological disorders and social distress associated with incapacitating incontinence as well as a sense of shame from the "deformity". Many patients with this disorder isolate themselves socially and suffer from anxiety and depression. [3-6] A nihilistic approach from both the patient and physicians may lead to delay in treatment, thus burdening the patient with years of suffering and diminished quality of life.

4. Diagnosis

A careful obstetric history and detailed physical exam of the perineal area is enough to make the diagnosis of traumatic cloaca. Inspection reveals the diminution or absence of the perineal body and the common genitourinary-gastrointestinal outlet. (Fig1, 2) A digital exam will reveal the length of the remaining anovaginal/rectovaginal septum as well as the relationship of the cervix with the rectum. This will aid in planning the appropriate surgical repair. The examining physician will also note a significant decrease in resting anal sphincter tone as well as a marked loss of voluntary squeeze pressure.

http://dx.doi.org/10.5772/57377

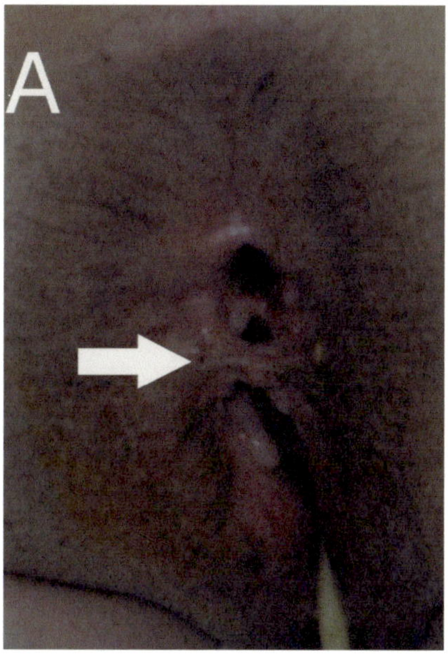

Figure 1. Traumatic cloaca with small bridge of skin between anus and vagina.

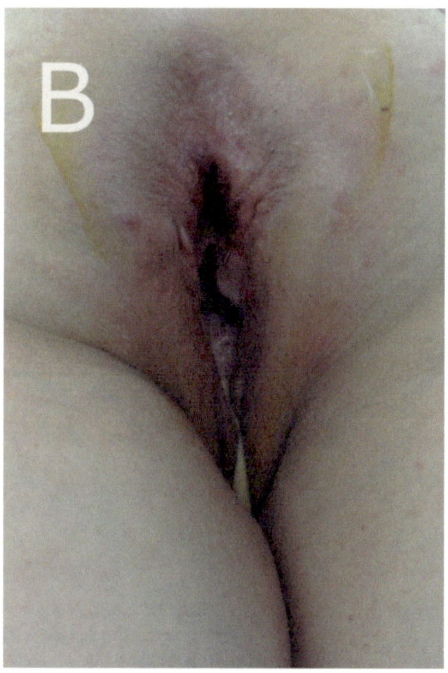

Figure 2. Traumatic cloaca. Note the incomplete anovaginal septum.

Additional diagnostic tests can be performed but are not mandatory. Endoanal ultrasound can be utilized to define the degree of the external and internal anal sphincter defect. In most cases, a significant defect of the anterior portion of both sphincters is present. Anal physiologic testing such as manometry documents the decrease in resting tone and squeeze pressure. Improvement in these parameters can be assessed after surgical repair of traumatic cloaca. Finally, transanal pudendal nerve stimulation provides evaluation of the neuromuscular integrity of the pelvic floor. [11] Pudendal nerve terminal motor latency can be used to predict the success of sphincteroplasty in incontinent patients with anterior sphincter defects. [12] Assessment of fecal incontinence can be performed with any number of validated tests such as the Cleveland Clinic Florida-Wexner Score or the St. Marks' incontinence score. [1, 13]

5. Treatment

Women with a traumatic cloaca defect are incapacitated in many aspects. Severe incontinence may lead to social isolation. Sexual dysfunction may result in depression and other psychological disorders. Both the patient and the obstetrician may be unaware that such defects can be repaired; therefore, traumatic cloaca may go untreated for many years.

The mainstay of conservative treatment is manipulation of stool consistency and frequency. This is done with fiber bulking and constipating medication such as loperamide. While this type of therapy is valid, results are not satisfactory. The anatomic defects that are associated with traumatic cloaca are such that severe incontinence persists despite conservative therapy. Surgical correction is usually necessary.

6. Surgical treatment

A variety of surgical techniques have been utilized to repair traumatic cloaca.

Surgical correction of these defects invariably involves the following steps:

1. Separation of the anorectum from the vagina by dissecting the rectovaginal septum.
2. Performance of an overlapping sphincteroplasty using both the external and internal anal sphincter, thus repairing the anterior defect.
3. Reconstruction of the perineal body by plicating the puborectalis muscle to the midline and skin closure.

6.1. Perineoplasty with X-flaps

This surgical technique was originally described by Corman [6] and was used both for traumatic cloaca repair as well as rectovaginal fistula repair. It is the technique most commonly used at our institution.

Preoperatively, all patients are given a full bowel preparation. Intravenous broad-spectrum antibiotics are administered preoperatively and continued for 24 hours post-surgery. The procedure is performed under general anaesthesia and the patient is placed in the prone-jacknife position with the buttocks taped apart and a urinary catheter in place.

The planned incisions are marked on the skin, where an "X" is outlined across the perineum, intersecting at the point of the anovaginal septum. (Fig 3)

The skin incision is performed, and flaps are developed to the ischiorectal fossae bi-laterally. Dissection is then carried out in the ischiorectal fossa cephalad up to the level of the levator muscles. (Fig 4)

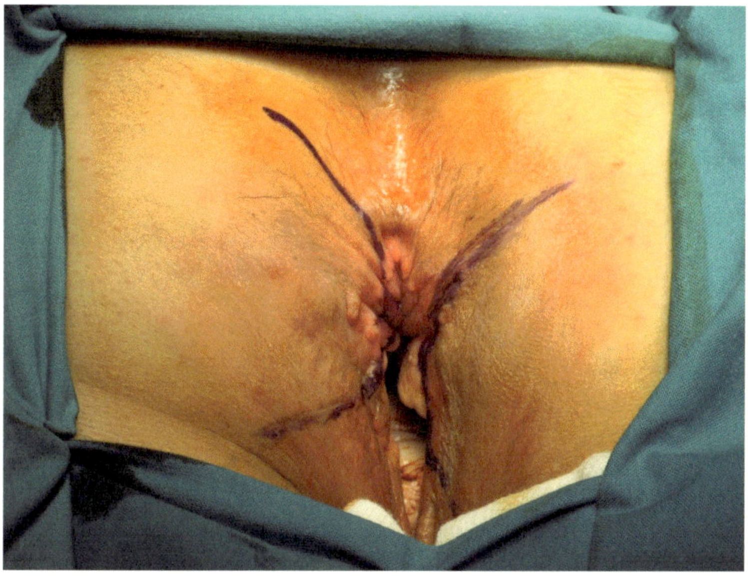

Figure 3. Outline of "X" incision on perineum.

The next step is division of the ano-vagial/rectovaginal septum. Initially, traction sutures are placed in the anal and vaginal mucosa. Then, the septum is divided with electrocautery, and dissection is carried out cephalad up to the level of the puborectalis muscle. (Fig 5) This division allows for mobilization of both the rectal and vaginal "tubes". During the following step, both edges of the sphincter complex are identified. Mobilization of the sphincter complex is performed lateral to medial. An overlapping sphincteroplasty was then done with interrupted sutures. At all times, a small retractor is placed in the anal canal, in order to prevent stenosis after repair. Midline approximation of the levators is performed with interrupted 2-0 poly-propylene sutures, thus filling the space between the anal and vaginal tubes and re-creating a perineal "body". Overlapping of the "X" flaps is then undertaken. The anterior wall of the anus and the posterior wall of the vagina are sutured to the skin of the newly constructed perineum. Layered closure with absorbable sutures is performed. (Fig 6) No drains are placed, and we do not routinely create a diverting stoma.

Postoperatively, betadine ointment is applied to the wounds daily. Metronidazole is given orally for 7 days. Patients are allowed moderate ambulation immediately; however, sitting is

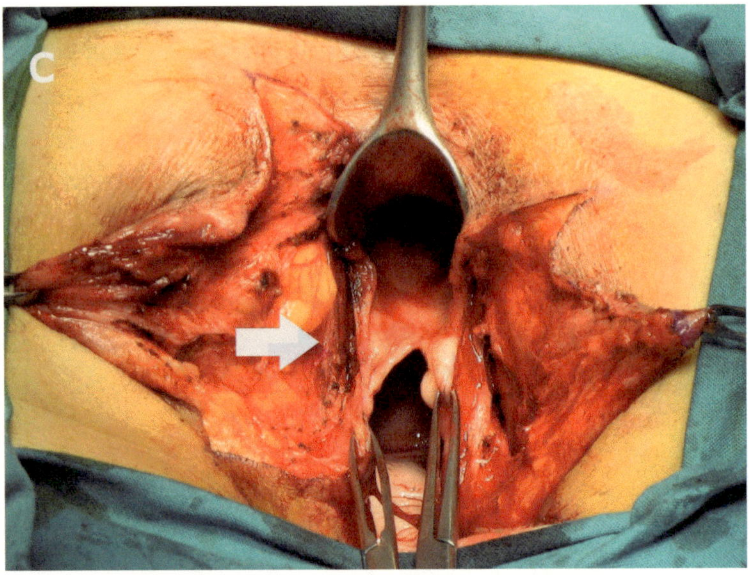

Figure 4. Flaps have been developed, and dissection up to the level of the puborectalis (arrow) is performed.

discouraged. Pharmacological bowel confinement is achieved by administering loperamide thrice daily for 5 days. A soft diet is started on the second postoperative day. Fiber supplements are given after discontinuation of loperamide.

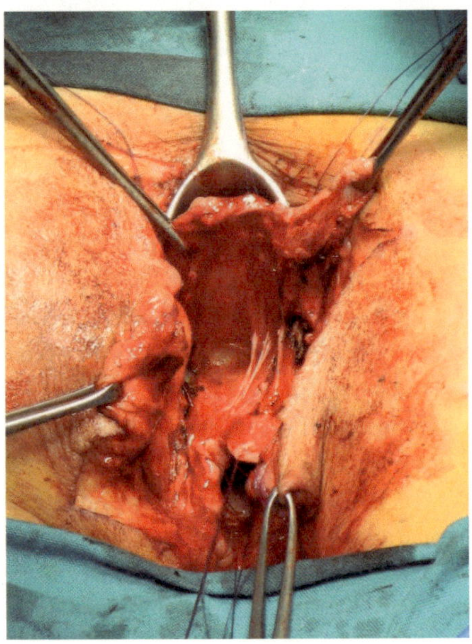

Figure 5. Divided anovaginal septum, with posterior vaginal wall superiorly.

http://dx.doi.org/10.5772/57377

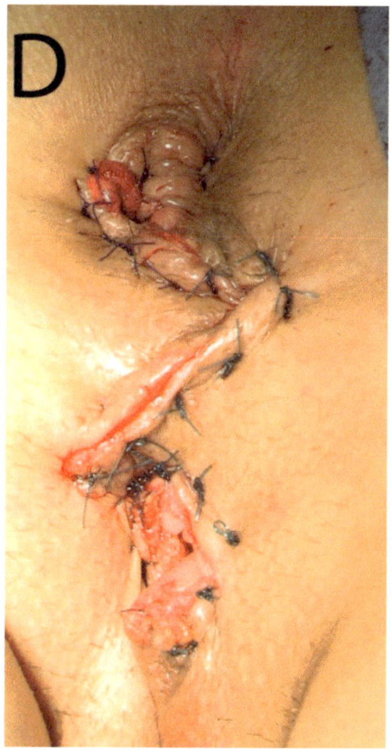

Figure 6. Completed repair, with separation of anus and vagina and restoration of perineal body.

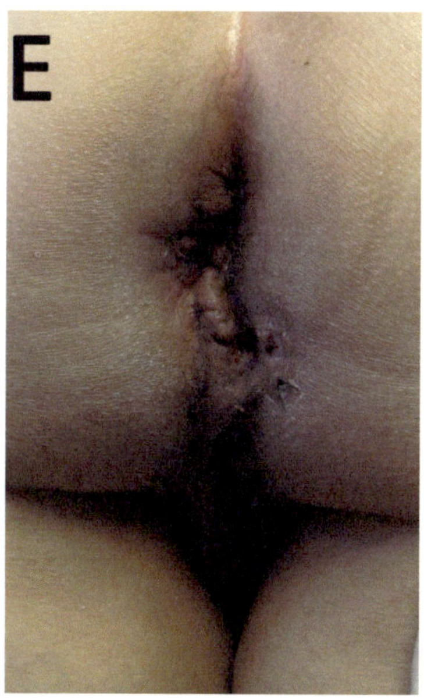

Figure 7. Repair at one month after surgical correction.

6.2. Transverse to vertical incision

An alternative technique, especially in patients with a low-profile perineum, (Fig 8) utilizes a transverse incision, made between the anus and vagina. This incision may also be curvilinear. Dissection of the ischiorectal fossae, division of the anovaginal septum, levatoroplasty and overlapping sphincteroplasty are performed in a fashion similar to the patients with the "X" flaps. The transverse incision is closed in a vertical fashion, thus creating a high-profile perineum. (Fig 9)

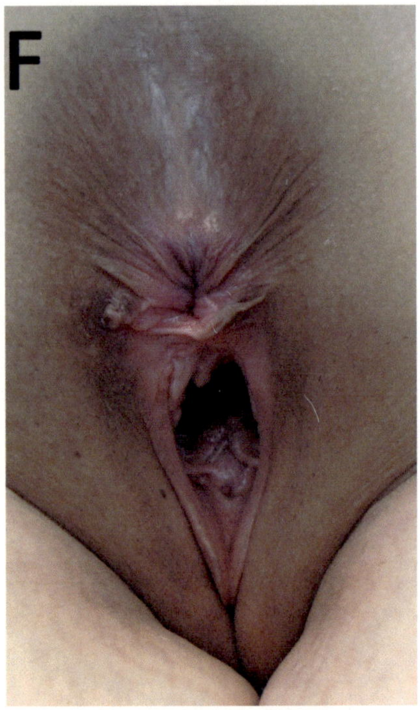

Figure 8. Patient with a low-profile perineum after obstetric injury. This patient underwent surgical correction utilizing a transverse-to vertical perineal incision.

6.3. Island flaps

Instead of primary closure of the skin, which is used in the techniques mentioned previously, perineal closure can be achieved by using island skin flaps.

Draganic and Solomon have reported their experience with island flap perineoplasty and concluded that wound dehiscence was significantly lower when skin flaps rather than simple wound approximation was used for perineal closure. [7] In their series, they performed a faecal diversion in 75% of their patients.

http://dx.doi.org/10.5772/57377

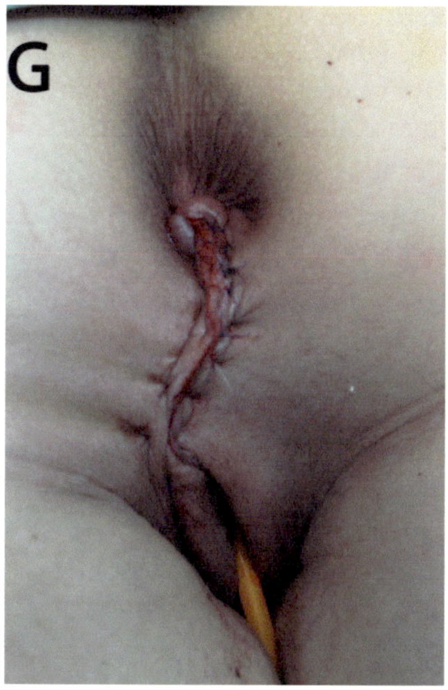

Figure 9. Postoperative photo of patient in previous figure. Result after vertical closure of incision, with restoration of perineal body.

7. Results of surgical correction

Despite the variety of techniques used in the correction of traumatic cloacal deformities, data on the outcome of these procedures is limited. Most reports are based on small series of patients; meta-analyses regarding results have not been performed.

The largest series of patients utilizing X-flaps for traumatic cloaca correction has been reported by Kaiser [4]. Twelve patients underwent this procedure in a 5-year period. No prophylactic diverting stomas were constructed. Three patients experienced postoperative rectovaginal fistula, and in one of these patients a stoma was necessary. Minor wound complications were observed in 8 patients. After surgical follow-up of 9.83 ± 2.8 months and long-term follow-up of 38.9 ± 6.9 months, all the patients were satisfied with regards to overall function, continence and cosmetic result.

In our own small series of 4 patients, mean hospital length stay was 5 ± 0.8 days (range 4-6). All patients were followed in the outpatient clinic weekly for the first month, then monthly for the next 3 months. Median follow-up was 27 months (range 10 – 52 months). One patient developed a small, superficial separation of the corner of the X-flap. This was resolved by placing sutures. One patient experienced significant constipation at 2 weeks postoperatively. This was treated with manual disimpaction and subsequent small-volume enemas. There were no wound infections, separation of the sphincter repair, or rectovaginal fistulas. At 1 month post-repair there was excellent healing of all wounds. (Fig 7)

At the latest follow-up visit, all patients reported significant improvement in fecal continence. The mean Cleveland Clinic Florida/Wexner score decreased from a mean preoperative value of 18.25 ± 0.95 to a postoperative value of 1.25 ±1.5. All patients required fibre supplement to maintain stool consistency. None of the patients required use of pads, and major incontinence episodes were ameliorated.

Regarding sexual activity, all patients were empirically advised to resume vaginal intercourse 3 months after repair. All patients resumed activity; one patient complained of dyspareunia at the end of the follow-up period.

Venkatesh and Ramanujam [3] reported surgical correction of traumatic cloaca in 44 patients over a 14-year period. The technique involved approximation of the internal and external sphincters together with the transverse perineal muscles in a vest-over- pants manner. The transverse perineal incision was closed vertically. The authors reported excellent functional results with minimal morbidity. A diverting stoma was not performed. Dyspareunia was reported in 27% of patients.

Excellent functional results have been also reported by Abcarian et al. [2] Their group performed surgical correction in 43 patients. Anal physiological testing was done preoperatively and postoperatively; most parameters (resting tone and voluntary squeeze pressures) return to normal after surgery.

Hollingshead et al reported on their experience in repairing traumatic cloacal deformities. [1] Twenty-nine patients underwent surgical repair over a 14-year period. The technique employed a curvilinear incision, division of the anovaginal septum, identification and mobilization of the cut sphincter edges. Then the anorectal defect was closed, a sphincteroplasty performed and the vagina repaired. In this series, the puborectalis or levator muscles were not plicated, and the initial incision was closed longitudinally. A stoma was constructed in 13 patients. Two out of 12 patients in whom a stoma was not fashioned at the time of repair developed a rectovaginal fistula and required subsequent bowel defunctioning. In most patients, improvement in incontinence scores, anophysiologic testing and sexual function.

8. Discussion

Traumatic cloacal deformities are rare post-obstetric injuries characterized by diminution or disruption of the perineal body, anterior division and lateral retraction of the anal sphincters, and loss of the distal ano/rectovaginal septum of varying length. [1-6]

These deformities may be a result of a third or fourth degree perineal laceration, which may or may not have been repaired. Failure of repair may be a result of hematoma, infection or technical mishaps. Partial failure may result in a rectovaginal fistula; complete failure leads to a cloacal deformity. [8]

Most, if not all patients have complete loss of defecatory control. This leads to skin irritation, genitourinary infections and a significant degree of sexual dysfunction.

The effect on the quality of life of these patients is profound. Patients feel "deformed", and may isolate themselves. Medical advice may be deferred for years. On the other hand, physicians may be unaware of the possibility of repair of such lesions and fail to refer to a specialist.

Conservative measures and/or pharmacologic manipulation of bowel movements do not improve quality of life and is not a sustainable treatment modality for this condition. Surgical treatment is required.

As in our small series, other authors have reported prior attempts to repair either a perineal laceration or a cloacal deformity before definitive correction. [2, 4] The timing of this definitive repair is extremely important. Early surgical repair may lead to failure as a result of active inflammation and absence of dissection planes. Therefore, most experts advise a waiting time of at least 3 months after index injury or previous repair before correction is undertaken. [2, 6]

Even though these lesions are rare, a variety of surgical techniques for correction have been described. [2-7] Most employ overlapping sphincteroplasty and division of the rectovaginal septum. Perineal body construction is performed in several ways. Closure at right angles to the original incision is one of the most common modes of perineal reconstruction. Others use island flaps or lotus petal flaps. [7, 10] Some authors advise partial closure of the wound, as to avoid wound infection, which is the most serious complication of cloacal repair. [2, 9]

Anovaginal and perineal reconstruction utilizing X flaps was initially described by Corman. [6] Kaiser reported a series of 12 patients in which improvement in fecal continence and sexual function was significant. [4] Possible downsides of this technique in comparison with others are the intrinsic complexity of the operation and potential problems with wound healing, specifically ischemia of the flaps. On the other hand, partial closure of a perineal wound may take time to heal, and may require multiple dressing changes and visits to clinic.

We believe the most important technical point in correction of cloacal deformities is the division of the anovaginal/rectovaginal septum, with mobilization of the anorectal and vaginal tubes. Herein lays the potential for failure of the repair. Several points regarding this division are important.

Firstly, meticulous hemostasis is mandatory. The vagina is an extremely vascular anatomical structure; large vessels (especially veins) surround it. A fair amount of bleeding may be encountered during anovaginal separation if an incorrect plane is entered. Hematoma formation with potential infection and abscess formation may lead to catastrophic results. Second, care should be taken not to "buttonhole" either the anorectum or vagina during this dissection. Unrepaired perforations in either structure may also lead to septic collections and failure of the operation. Third, interposition of tissue in the space created by the division must be utilized. This constructs a perineal body and supports the sphincteroplasty. It also fills dead space and eliminates the possibility of fluid collections, which, as mentioned before, may lead to failure. Plication of the puborectalis muscle seems to be the easiest choice of tissue for this interposition, since it is in immediate anatomical proximity. Other potential techniques should the puborectalis prove to be inadequate, are utilization of a bulbocarvernosus (Martius) flap, or a gracilis muscle flap. This could add significant complexity to the repair, however.

Some authors advocate construction of a temporary stoma. [1, 10] Proponents of fecal diversion maintain that this allows accelerated perineal healing and avoidance of infection and failure of the repair. The mechanics of defecation in the immediate perioperative period may also potentially lead to disruption of the puborectalis plication or other tissue interposition. Stomas are associated with significant morbidity (skin irritation, prolapse, hernia), and need a second operation for closure. [8, 9] In addition, they do not seem to improve outcomes. Some experts reserve diversion for major failure of the perineal repair. [3, 4]

The most common complications reported after correction of traumatic cloacal deformities are minor wound infection, rectovaginal fistula and breakdown of the perineal wound. These may occur in up to 40% of cases [1]. Expectant therapy and revision of repair are utilized in these instances [1, 4]

After definitive correction of traumatic cloacal deformities, sexual activity and subsequent pregnancies should be deferred; however, the exact "safe" time period remains to be determined. Some authors advise sexual abstinence for at least 6 weeks post repair. [8] Caesarean section after complex perineal repairs seems reasonable.

Finally, improvement in fecal incontinence is significant following cloacal repair in most series even after long-term follow-up. [1, 3, 4].

9. Conclusion — Summary

Traumatic cloacal deformities are the least frequent complications of obstetric injuries to the anorectum. Repair and reconstruction of all anatomical structures involved is feasible with satisfactory cosmetic and functional results. Correction of these deformities can be performed using a variety of techniques. Careful dissection and division of the anovaginal/rectovaginal septum is a crucial step in the creation of a new perineal body. Referral to a specialist colorectal surgeon familiar with repair of traumatic cloacal deformities may improve the quality of life of patients. Fecal diversion is not mandatory.

Author details

Constantine P. Spanos*

Address all correspondence to: costasspanos@hotmail.com

Department of Surgery, Aristotelian University, Thessaloniki, Greece

References

[1] Hollingshead JRF, Warusavitarne J, Vaizey CJ, Northover JMA. Outcomes following repair of traumatic cloacal deformities. Br J Surg 2009;96:1082-1085

http://dx.doi.org/10.5772/57377

[2] Abcarian H, Orsay CP, Pearl RK, et al. Traumatic cloaca. Dis Colon Rectum 1989;32:783-787

[3] Venkatesh KS, Ramanujam P. Surgical treatment of traumatic cloaca. Dis Colon Rectum 1996;39:811-816

[4] Kaiser AM. Cloaca-like deformity with fecal incontinence after after severe obstetric injury-technique and functional outcome of ano-vaginal and perineal reconstruction with X-flaps and sphincteroplasty. Colorectal Dis 2008;10:827-832

[5] Mercês RL, Pisi PH, Balestrim Fo A, et al. Surgical treatment of traumatic cloaca. Acta Cir Bras 2008; 23 Suppl 1, 1:105-107

[6] Corman, ML. Anal incontinence following obstetrical injury. Dis Colon Rectum 1985;28 :86-89

[7] Draganic B, Solomon MJ. Island flap perineoplasty for coverage of perineal skin defects after repair of cloacal deformity. ANZ J Surg 2001;71:487-490

[8] Spanos CP, Mikos T, Kastanias E, et al. Surgical treatment of traumatic cloaca. Arch Gynecol Obstet 2012;286:815-818

[9] Valente MA, Khanduja KS. Layered surgical repair of traumatic cloacal deformities: technical details and functional outcomes. Tech Coloproctol 2012; 16:153-156

[10] Altomare DF, Rinaldi M, Bucaria V, et al. Overlapping sphincteroplasty and modified lotus petal flap for delayed repair of traumatic cloaca. Tech Coloproctol 2007; 11:268-270

[11] Kiff ES, Swash M. Slowed conduction in the pudendal nerves in idiopathic (neurogenic) fecal incontinence. Br J Surg 1984; 71:614-16

[12] Wexner SD, Marchetti F, Jagelman DG. The role of sphincteroplasty for fecal incontinence reevaluated: prospective physiologic and functional review. Dis Colon Rectum 1996; 39:1164-70

[13] Jorge JM, Wexner SD. Etiology and management of fecal incontinence. Dis Colon Rectum 1993; 36:77-97

Chapter 10

Medical and Surgical Management of Fecal Incontinence after Repair of High Imperforate Anus Anomalies

Talal Abdallah Al-Malki

Additional information is available at the end of the chapter

1. Introduction

Fecal incontinence is a socially distressing misfortunate condition, which can be very embarrassing. It affects children, with dramatic behavioral and personality changes, with patients becoming socially withdrawn and reluctant to leave their homes. Victims are housebound and become socially disruptive. This condition may be due to (1) congenital anorectal malformations (2) trauma to anal sphincter (3) injuries to the sphincter following operations on the anal canal and (4) central nervous disease or nerve injury.

It can occur from a variety of conditions. The most common is overflow incontinence from functional fecal retention, but it can also occur in otherwise healthy children with functional nonretentive fecal soiling or in children with organic causes of fecal incontinence, such as congenital malformations, or any other condition affecting the anorectum, anal sphincters, or the spinal cord.

Mild to moderate incontinence, when there is no injury to the sphincters, can be treated by dietary modification, pharmacological treatment and behavioral therapy. Dietary modification entails having foods with high fiber content such as fruits, vegetables, beans and whole wheat bread. Pharmacological treatment includes prescription of synthetic cellulose and psyllium husk derived from the plantago tree, and antidiarrhea drugs such as Loperamide, diphenoxylate hydrochloride and codeine phosphate. Behavioral therapy techniques involve toilet training; urge control strategies, as well as pelvic floor physical therapy and biofeedback.

Surgical management of fecal incontinence should be reserved for patients with identifiable anal sphincter defects. It includes sphincteroplasty, which is indicated for sphincter disruption after surgical procedures, and muscle transpositions procedures, that are recommended when anal incontinence is secondary to anal sphincter disruption unresponsive to repair, neurogenic sphincter compromise, or congenital sphincter disorders. Muscle transpositions procedures include graciloplasty and gluteoplasty.

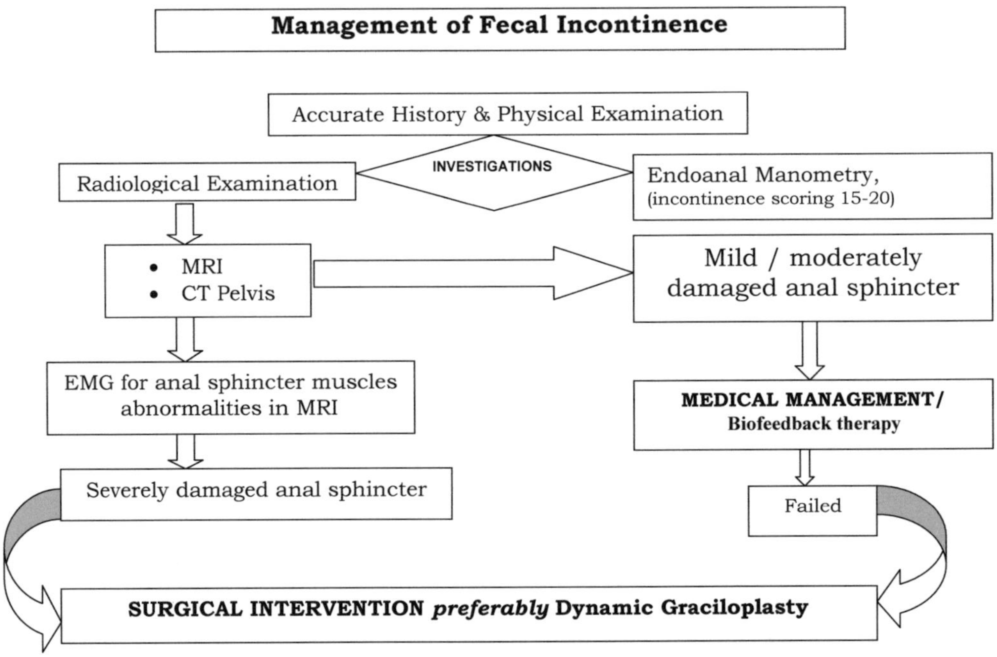

2. Medical and surgical managementof fecal incontinence

Graciloplasty was first described in 1952 by Pickrell who carried out gracilis muscle transposition for management in the pediatric population. The majority of muscle fibers in the gracilis are type II fast twitch, easily fatigable as opposed to approximately 80% of type I slow twitch, fatigue resistant muscle fibers in the external anal sphincter. Beaten and his coworkers introduced neurostimulation of the gracilis with the idea of converting type II muscle fibers to type I fatigue-resistant fibers (dynamic graciloplasty).

Other modalities for managing incontinence include artificial anal sphincter (Acticon Neosphincter™, American Medical Systems, Minnetonka, MN), which is indicated for patients with anal incontinence secondary to neurologic disorders that affect the sphincter muscles or trauma. This procedure is generally contraindicated in patients with severe diarrhea disorders, poor functional status, or physical and/or mental disease that would limit their ability to adequately use the artificial sphincter. The Secca procedure is another alternative for such patients, where temperature-controlled radio-frequency energy is delivered to the anal musculature through a specially designed anoscopic instrument. It offers a less-invasive option for treatment of fecal incontinence, as compared to surgery, and is performed on an outpatient

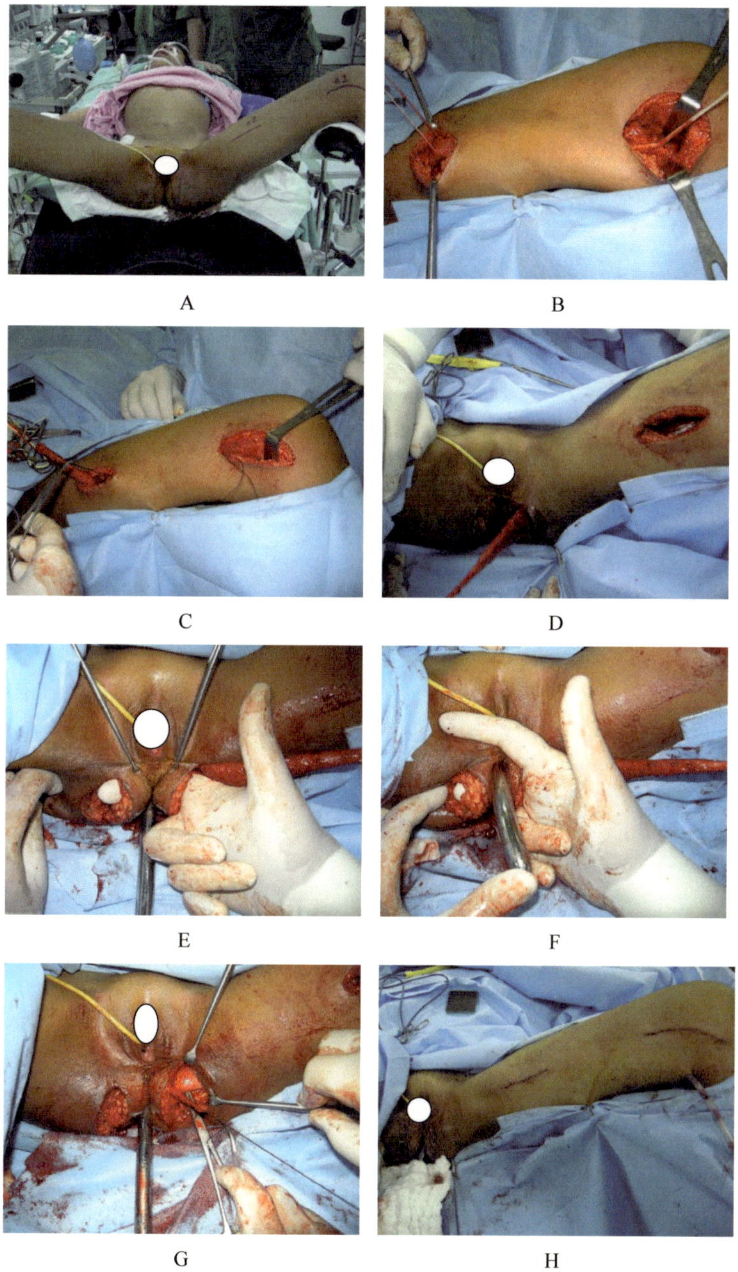

Figure 1. Dynamic graciloplasty in a fecal incontinence patient. The surgery was performed in all patients who failed to respond to all non surgical management, in addition to the cases that demonstrated bad condition of the external anal sphincter by MRI, EMG and Manometry. A: Incisions marks before Gracilis muscle dissection; B: Gracilis muscle completely dissected; C: Gracilis muscle pulled out of its bed; D: Gracilis muscle pulled out of its bed; E: tunneling above the anus; F: Gracilis muscle tunneling below the anus; G: Gracilis muscle wrapped around anal canal; H: Wound closed.

basis using conscious sedation. Sacral neuro-modulation is another modality for management; the procedure involves the placement of a quadrupolar electrode through the sacral foramina of S3 or S4 to stimulate the pelvic floor musculature. Injectable bulking agents have been used for anal incontinence that results secondary to internal anal sphincter incompetence or disruption. Autologous fat, collagen, Teflon paste and, most recently, injectable silicone particles and PTP (Bioplastique) have been used as bulking agents.

For all patients who undergo the procedure, thorough history taking including the nature of the congenital lesion and the type of surgical intervention should be preformed. The degree of incontinence is usually determined. Waxner and his co-workers graded fecal incontinence in children based on the type of fecal contents, need to wear pad and whether there is alteration in life style and the frequency of occurrence of the afore mentioned factors using a score with a range between 0 (never) and 20 (complete incontinence). Then a meticulous physical examination should be done, with special emphasis on the anal sphincter. Pelvic CT scanning and MRI should be executed to define the status of the sacrum and pelvis, and that of the sphincter complex. EMG for anal sphincter muscles should be performed in the cases that show abnormalities in MRI. Furthermore, anorectal manometry, is to be carried out to quantify the impact of sphincter injury on sphincter function by measures both resting anal sphincter canal tone (internal anal sphincter activity) and squeeze pressure (external sphincter activity) in four quadrants (anterior, right, left, and posterior).

For patients who exhibit severely damaged anal sphincter by MRI, EMG, and endoanal manometry, (incontinence scoring 15-20). These patients should be scheduled to surgery without giving trial to conservative management. The management approach, for other cases, should start with medical treatment and behavioral therapy. Patients who fail to respond properly should be subjected to surgery.

Patients should be instructed to increase dietary fiber contents. They should be told to collect 25-30 gms of dietary fiber per day.

Patients who fail to abide by the regimen should be given the fiber supplements methylcellulose and psyllium husk derived from the plantago tree. In cases with loose stool the antidiarrhea drug Loperamide hydrochloride should be prescribed.

In addition to the above dietary and medical management, behavioral techniques i.e. *Toileting techniques* and *Urge control* should be applied in all patients.

Patients who fail to respond to the above management protocol have to be sent to a biofeedback therapist. There they should be subjected to two types of training:

A motor part: This comprised insertion of an anal manometric probe which transform the contractions of the anal sphincter to a visual display, allowing the child to learn how to contract his sphincter properly in an increasing force to overcome fecal soiling.

A sensory part: A manometric balloon probe is to be inserted into the rectum; the balloon is filled with air to train the child to respond to the sensation of rectal filling.

Patients who are scheduled for surgical intervention are those who failed to respond to all non surgical management, in addition to the cases that demonstrated bad condition of the external anal sphincter by MRI, EMG and manometry.

The technique of graciloplasty is performed by using the left gracilis muscle. The muscle should be dissected till the neurovascular bundle entrance, tunneled and wrapped around the anal canal and sutured to itself using proline stitches. All wounds should be irrigated and closed; a suction drain is placed along the gracilis bed. Postoperatively, both lower limbs should be kept in adduction for three days.

Dynamic graciloplasty entails electric stimulation of the muscle after surgery to transform its fibers to type I slow twitch, fatigue resistant muscle fibers. Chronic low-frequency stimulation should be undertaken in six sessions at 2-week interval over the subsequent 12 weeks. During these sessions, the amount of time during which the muscle been stimulated is to be gradually increased until full-time stimulation is achieved. The conversion of the muscle could be seen in the decreased fusion frequency and the capacity of the muscle to sustain a prolonged contraction. When this status has been achieved, the muscle will show continuous contraction and the anal canal is expected to respond by continuous closure.

The primary step is to assess the degree of incontinence and degree of anal sphincter damage. This is done using a scoring system for incontinence, pelvic MRI, endoanal manometry and EMG. Although endoanal ultra-sonography is very effective to demonstrate the degree of anal sphincter injury, it is sometimes not performed due to the unavailability of an expert sonographer for interpretation of results. The decision taken, for children to be managed surgically from the start, is usually made based on the input from all investigations (continence score 15-20, damaged anal sphincter as illustrated by MRI, Manometry and EMG). Those cases that are treated medically with dietary management and medical treatment. Antidiarrheal drugs are to be used in cases with loose stool.

Patients not responding to medication should be sent to biofeedback therapy. Most cases are expected to show low compliance to the therapy and may refuse to complete the sessions. In general, it is expected that biofeedback in children is discouraging. However, it may show some improvement at early follow up, but not after long term follow up. It has been reported that even demonstrated higher rather than lower rates of persisting symptoms of fecal incontinence up to 12 months when biofeedback is added to conventional treatment. Biofeedback needs not only a skilled therapist, but in addition the will and determination of the patient; which is difficult to achieve in such young ages of patients.

Usually dynamic graciloplasty, is performed following the the conventional operative steps as described in literature. However, the gracilis tendon may be wrapped around the anus and been sutured to itself, instead of suturing it to the opposite ischial tuberosity. Furthermore, one gracilis muscle may be used for repair, while in some other reports both muscles were employed to form a sling around the anal canal simulating the action of the puborectalis. Nonetheless, no superior outcomes were demonstrated to have been achieved as compared to the technique adopted using the gracilis tendon wrapped around the anus. In the later technique short-and medium-term morbidity rates, are lower compared to the conventional techniques. Wound seroma that may take place in some cases in the bed of gracilis muscle, may be drained with complete cure outcomes. Wound infections can be managed and cured with drainage and antibiotics according to culture and sensitivity. Medium-term follow up is necessary for patients who may suffer anal stenosis, which is to be treated with a regular schedule of dilatation, and for cases that experience fecal impaction, disimpaction may be performed under anesthesia.

3. Conclusion

Children with low incontinence score (5-10) after repair of high imperforate anus anomalies, which show no evidence of anatomical damage of the sphincter, can be treated successfully with medical treatment, while Biofeedback therapy has discouraging results, because it is refused by children. Therefore, cases who fail medical treatment or have high incontinence score (16-20) are recommended to undergo surgical intervention preferably dynamic gracilo-plasty which proved 100% success rate and demonstrated excellent results in the operated children.

Author details

Talal Abdallah Al-Malki

College of Medicine, Taif University, Pediatric Surgery Department, Alhada Armed Forces Hospital, Taif, Kingdom of Saudi Arabia

References

[1] Pensabene L, Nurko S. Management of fecal incontinence in children without functional fecal retention. *Currt Treat Options Gastroenterol* 2004; 7:.381-390.

[2] Parker SC, Thorsen A. Fecal incontinence. *Surg Clin North Am* 2002; 82: 1273–1290.

[3] Scarlett Y. Medical management of fecal incontinence. *Gastroenterology* 2004; 126: S55–63.

[4] Rudolph W, Galandiuk S. A practical guide to the diagnosis and management of fecal incontinence. *Mayo Clin Proc* 2002; 77: 271–275.

[5] Norton C. Behavioral management of fecal incontinence in adults. *Gastroenterology* 2004; 126: S64–S70.

[6] Corman ML. Colon and Rectal Surgery.5th ed. Philadelphia: Lippincott Williams and Wilkins; 2004.

[7] Sielezneff I, Malouf AJ, Bartolo DC, Pryde A, Douglas S. Dynamic graciloplasty in the treatment of patients with fecal incontinence. *Br J Surg* 1999; 86: 61–65.

[8] Christiansen J, Hansen CR, Rasmussen O. Bilateral gluteus maximus transposition for anal incontinence. *Br J Surg* 1995; 82:903–905.

[9] Pickrell KL, Broadbent TR, Masters FW, Metzger JT. Construction of a rectal sphincter and restoration of anal continence by transplanting the gracilis muscle; a report of four cases in children. *Ann Surg* 1952; 135: 853–862.

[10] Williams NS, Hallan RI, Koeze TH, Pilot MA, Watlens ES. Construction of a neoanal sphincter by transposition of the gracilis and prolonged neuromuscular stimulation for the treatment of fecal incontinence. *Ann R Coll Surg Engl* 1990; 72: 108-113.

[11] Baeten CG, Bailey HR, Bakka A, Belliveau P, Berg E, Buie WD et al. Safety and efficacy of dynamic graciloplasty for fecal incontinence: report of a prospective, multicenter trial. Dynamic Graciloplasty Therapy Study Group. *Dis Colon Rectum* 2000; 43: 743–751

[12] Madoff RD, Baeten CG, Christiansen J, Rosen HR, Williams NS, Heine JA. Standards for anal sphincter replacement. *Dis Colon Rectum* 2000; 43: 135–141.

[13] Takahashi T, Garcia-Osogobio S, Valdovinos MA, Belmonte C, Barreto C, Velasco L. Extended two-year results of radio-frequency energy delivery for the treatment of fecal incontinence (the Secca procedure). *Dis Colon Rectum* 2003; 46: 711–715.

[14] Matzel KE, Stadelmaier U, Hohenfellner M, Gall FP. Electrical stimulation of sacral spinal nerves for treatment of fecal incontinence. *Lancet* 1995; 346:1124–1127.

[15] Tjandra JJ, Lim JF, Hiscock R, Rajendra P. Injectable silicone biomaterial for fecal incontinence caused by internal anal sphincter dysfunction is effective. *Dis Colon Rectum.* 2004; 47: 2138–2146.

[16] Blaisdell PC. Repair of the incontinent sphincter ani. *Am J Surg* 1957; 94: 573-576.

[17] Rudolph W, Galandiuk S. A practical Guide to the Diagnosis and Management of Fecal Incontinence. *Mayo Clin Proc* 2002; 77: 271-275.

[18] Loening-Baucke V. Modulation of abnormal defecation dynamics by biofeedback treatment in chronically constipated children with encopresis. *J Pediatr* 1990; 116: 214-222.

[19] Loening-Baucke V. Biofeedback treatment for chronic constipation and encopresis in childhood: long-term outcome. *Pediatrics* 1995; 96: 105-110.

[20] Brazelli M, Griffiths P. Behavioural and cognitive interventions with or without other treatments for the management of fecal incontinence in children. *Cochrane Database of Systematic Reviews* 2006; 19: CD002240.

[21] Nixon HH. Operation for incontinence following anorectal anomalies: Levatorplasty and gracilis transplantation. Rob and Smith's Operative Surgery colon, rectum and anus. 5th ed. Chapman and Hill; 1993: 460-461.

[22] Madoff RD, Rosen HR, Baeten CG, LaFontaine LJ, Cavina E, Devesa M. Safety and efficacy of dynamic muscle plasty for anal incontinence: lessons from a prospective, multicenter trial. *Gastroenterology* 1999;116: 549-556.

[23] Thornton MJ, Kennedy ML, Lubowski DZ, King DW. Long-term follow-up of dynamic graciloplasty for fecal incontinence. *Colorectal Dis* 2004; 6: 470-476.

[24] Wexner SD, Gonzalez-Padron A, Teoh TA, Moon HK. The stimulated gracilis neosphincter for fecal incontinence: a new use for an old concept. *Plast Reconsr Surg* 98; 1996: 693-699

[25] Wright JJr, Gehrich AP, Albright TS. Mangement of Anal Incontinence. *J Pelvic Med Surg* 12; 2006: 125-140

Chapter 11

Long Term Outcome After Surgery for Anorectal Malformation

Anthony G. Catto-Smith, Misel Trajanovska and Russell Taylor

Additional information is available at the end of the chapter

http://dx.doi.org/10.5772/57072

1. Introduction

Anorectal malformations (ARM) are a spectrum of congenital caudal end defects affecting the normal development of the anus and rectum that are usually easily detected after birth by physical examination. They are relatively common, occurring in approximately 1 in 5,000 live births, and vary markedly in severity. ARM is frequently associated with other congenital anomalies that may have a much more severe impact on long-term prognosis [1]. ARM are classified into low, intermediate and high subtypes depending on the relationship of the defect to the pelvic floor musculature [2]. A variety of surgical procedures have been developed for their correction, but despite this faecal incontinence is a well-recognized long-term complication that is said to occur in between 10% to 33% or more of patients with ARM [3-6].

Most reviews of outcome after surgical repair of ARM grade continence into broad classifications of "good", "fair" or "poor", based on scoring systems developed by Kelly [7], Templeton [5], Kiesewetter [8] or Wingspread [9]. Faecal incontinence has a significant impact on quality of life in both children and adults [10]. These classification systems have been crucially important in providing statistical information about incontinence but provide little help in understanding how and when incontinence occurs, and its impact at an individual level.

The aims of our study were to define the extent, severity and types of faecal incontinence in children after surgical repair of anorectal malformations, as well as its impact on health care usage, medication, dietary intake, and quality of life. We also wished to relate these outcomes to the level of abnormality, whether "high", "intermediate" or "low".

2. Methods

2.1. Ethical approval

Ethical approval for this study was obtained from the Ethics in Human Research Committee of the Royal Children's Hospital (Approval number EHRC 21118B)

2.2. Subjects

We planned to recruit all patients who had presented for treatment of anorectal malformations to the Royal Children's Hospital, Melbourne between 1974 and 2001. Subjects were identified through ICD coding of medical records. We included patients coded with the diagnoses of anorectal agenesis, rectal atresia, anal agenesis, anorectal stenosis (1970-80; ICD 751.30-33); colonic atresia and stenosis, imperforate anus, anorectal agenesis, anal agenesis (1981-88; ICD 751.20-23); atresia and stenosis of large intestine, rectum and anal canal (1989-2002; ICD-10-AM, 751.2, q42.1-3, q42.18, q 43.6).

We excluded those who were deceased, or non-English speaking, or permanently resident overseas. Clinical information was obtained from medical records. Patients were sub-divided into either a combined high and intermediate category or a low malformation category based on coding information. We also inspected operative notes and separately confirmed correct classification of the level of malformation using the Wingspread Conference criteria [11]. Most patients had the same classification irrespective of the method used. Discrepancies between the two were resolved after inspection of the notes by a paediatric surgeon (RGT).

Recruitment packs were mailed to the most current address recorded in the hospital records. Each recruitment pack contained a detailed information sheet about the study and an initial consent form to allow further discussion of the project. Upon receipt of the signed consent form, we contacted each subject or parent by phone to provide further detailed information about the project and to schedule a detailed interview to administer a structured questionnaire.

2.3. Questionnaire and diary

The 70-item questionnaire was administered either in person, by phone or by mail. The questionnaire had been modified from previous studies on outcome after surgical repair of Hirschsprung disease [12-14]. The revised questionnaire incorporated more detailed information related to bowel function, including amount and awareness of soiling as well as constipation. Further questions were included which related to physical and social functioning, current provision of health care and general health status. The questionnaire was further modified to enable it to be completed by patients as well as parents.

The revised questionnaire was piloted on 21 patients with Hirschsprung's disease. No significant further modifications were required.

Following the interview, respondents were asked to complete a four-week diary detailing bowel habit, faecal soiling, abdominal pain, enuresis and any medical therapy. This was also based on the diary used for the previous study [12]. Soiling was classified into two groups ("light" and "heavy") using the amount and frequency of episode. "Heavy" soiling was classified as being larger than a streak (able to be scraped from underclothing) and occurring at least once a month. "Light" soiling was classified as being no larger than a streak (unable to be scraped from underclothing) and occurring less than once a month. Functional testing, including anorectal manometry and electromyography, was offered [15].

Data from patients who had Down's syndrome was analysed separately.

2.4. Statistics

Statistical analysis was performed using SPSS version 12.0 (Statistical Package for the Social Sciences). Where appropriate, we used t-test, One-Way ANOVA, Chi-square or Fisher's Exact test, Mann-Whitney U Test or Kruskal-Wallis Test. Results were considered significant if $p<0.05$. Data are reported as mean ± standard deviation. Patients who were still in nappies because they were too young to be toilet trained were excluded from some analyses. Missing data are reflected in *n* values.

3. Results

353 patients were identified from ICD coding. We excluded 21 patients for whom we could not obtain permission from the treating surgeon. This was primarily because these surgeons were no longer in practice and had the effect of reducing the number of older patients. A further 34 patients were excluded who were deceased, 2 from overseas, 2 who needed an interpreter and 8 with inadequate contact details. 286 recruitment packs were mailed. Of these, 67 were returned by the post office with "wrong address" and no forwarding details, and no responses were obtained from a further 110 patients. 35 respondents declined or were unable to participate in the study. 74 respondents agreed to participate in the study, of whom 67 were interviewed. Two of the interviewed patients were later excluded because of an incorrect diagnosis. 57 were interviewed over the phone, 7 face to face and 1 via mailed questionnaires. Three patients had Down's syndrome.

The average age of the 62 interviewed patients without Down's was 11.4 ± 6.4yr; 41 were male and 21 female. The average age of the patients who were presumed to be alive but not interviewed was 18.2 ± 8.4yr of whom 428 were male and 275 female. Interviewed patients were younger ($p<0.001$) but gender proportions were similar ($p=0.59$). Four patients who wore nappies were excluded from some analyses. Two wore nappies only overnight (mean age 5.2 ± 1.6yr) and two were too young to be toilet trained, wearing nappies both day and night (mean age 2.4 ± 0.1yr).

12 patients underwent anorectal manometry and electromyography.

Clinical Data (n=62) (Table 1)

There were 28 patients with high/intermediate and 34 with low anorectal malformations. Both groups were similar in age, occupational prestige and family status. Eight patients who had developed significant faecal incontinence had undergone redo posterior sagittal ano-recto-plasty (PSARP) [16]. Of these, seven had high/intermediate malformations. Patients with high/intermediate malformations were more likely to have co-morbidity.

HD	High/Intermediate (n=28)	Low (n=34)	p	Total
Age (years)	11.8 ± 6.2	11.1 ± 6.7	0.65	11.4 ± 6.4
Gender	21M:7F	20M:14F	0.18	41M:21F
Daniel Occupational Prestige Score	4.4 ± 1.0	4.3 ± 0.9	0.81	4.4 ± 1.0
Single Parent Family n (%) n=62	7 (11.5)	7 (11.5)	0.68	14 (23)
Co-morbidities n (%) n=62	21 (34)	15 (24)	0.01	36 (58)
Subsequent PSARP	7 (87.5)	1 (12.5)	0.02	8 (100)

Table 1. Clinical Data for interviewed patients.

Bowel Habit (n=60) (Table 2)

Patients with a past history of either high/intermediate or low malformations passed a similar number of bowel actions each week (5.5 ± 1.8). Patients with a history of PSARP had more bowel actions each week, although this just failed to reach statistical significance (PSARP 6.6 ± 1.1 vs no PSARP 5.3 ± 1.8, p=0.052). Patients with high/intermediate malformations were more likely to have a looser (liquid or pasty) stool consistency.

		High / Intermediate	Low	p	Total
Bowel actions per week		5.9 ± 1.6	5.2 ± 1.9	0.13	5.5 ± 1.9
Stool consistency n (%)					
	Liquid	3 (10.7)	1 (3.1)		4 (6.7)
	Pasty	11 (39.3)	6 (18.8)		17 (28.3)
	Formed	7 (25)	21 (65.6)		28 (46.7)
	Variable	7 (25)	4 (12.5)	0.01	11 (18.3)

Table 2. Bowel habit data for interviewed patients.

Faecal Continence (n=57) (Table 3)

Impairment in sensation of impending stool was common (38%), as was faecal urgency (74%), difficulty in holding back stool (40%) or controlling flatus (48%) and discriminating stool type (33%).

Patients with high/intermediate malformations were more likely to have difficulty sensing impending stool and holding it back. Younger patients were more likely to experience episodes of faecal urgency (urgency: young 0-11yr 30/36 vs old 12-33yr 12/21, p<0.05). Patients were more likely to have had episodes of faecal soiling during the last year when they also reported problems with sensation, holding back stool, urgency and stool discrimination. (Impaired sensation of impending stool: soiling 17/35 vs no soiling 3/26, $p<0.05$; inability to hold back stool: soiling 22/38 vs no soiling 0/15, $p<0.001$; faecal urgency: soiling 34/42 vs no soiling 8/15, $p<0.05$; or problems with stool discrimination: soiling 14/30 vs no soiling 1/14, $p<0.05$).

		High/Intermediate n (%)	Low n (%)	p	Total n (%)
Sensation impending stool (n=53)	Never/Rarely/Sometimes	15 (62.5)	5 (17.2)		20 (37.7)
	Often/Always	9 (37.5)	24 (82.8)	0.00	33 (62.3)
Faecal urgency (n=57)	Yes	17 (65.4)	25 (80.6)	0.19	42 (73.7)
Faecal urgency – frequency (n=36)	Rarely/Sometimes	9 (69.2)	12 (52.2)		21 (58.3)
	Often/Always	4 (30.8)	11 (47.8)	0.32	15 (41.7)
Ability to hold back stool (n=55)	Never/Rarely/Sometimes	14 (53.8)	8 (27.6)		22 (40)
	Often/Always	12 (46.2)	21 (72.4)	0.05	33 (60)
If able to hold back stool – how long? (n=44)	Seconds	4 (21.0)	2 (8)		6 (13.6)
	Couple minutes	12 (63.2)	16 (64)		28 (63.6)
	Greater than 30 mins	3 (15.8)	7 (28)	0.38	10 (22.7)
Discriminates stool consistencies (n=45)	Never/Sometimes	9 (45)	6 (24)		15 (33.3)
	Always	11 (55)	19 (76)	0.14	30 (66.7)
Stool discrimination type (n=34)	Formed & liquid	0 (-)	1 (5.3)		1 (2.9)
	Formed & gaseous	12 (80)	11 (57.9)		23 (67.7)
	Formed & liquid & gaseous	3 (20)	7 (36.8)	0.36	10 (29.4)
Uncontrolled flatus (n=29)	Never/Rarely/Sometimes	7 (50)	8 (53.3)	0.86	15 (51.7)
	Often / Always	7 (50)	7 (46.7)		14 (48.3)

Table 3. Continence data for interviewed patients.

Most patients (44/60, 73%) had soiling accidents at least once in the past year and this happened "often or always" in 22. 24 soiled only during the day and 20 soiled both during the day and overnight. There were none who soiled only at night. A higher proportion of females reported soiling episodes (female 19/21 vs male 25/39, p<0.05). 43 patients were able to quantify the usual size of soiling episodes that occurred during the daytime. This was medium to large in 26 (60%). Of the 18 who were able to describe the consistency of daytime soiling, 9 (50%) indicated that it was pasty. Eleven had episodes of daytime soiling but were usually unaware that these were occurring (more than 75% of the time). Nocturnal soiling was of pasty consistency in 60% (3/5) patients and medium to large amount in 43% (6/14).

Patients with a past history of high/intermediate malformations were more likely to "often or always" soil during the daytime than those with low malformations (soiling often/always: high/intermediate 15/28 vs low 7/31, p<0.05). Despite their revision, those with a PSARP still soiled more frequently (soiling often/always: PSARP 7/8 vs no PSARP 15/51, p<0.01). They were also more likely to soil at night (soiling often/always: PSARP 2/7 vs no PSARP 1/48, p<0.05).

Most patients could be classified as having either heavy or light soiling based upon frequency and amount of episodes. Nine patients (daytime soiling 1, nocturnal soiling 9) were unable to accurately define the amount or frequency of their soiling episodes. A third (12/33) of patients had "heavy" soiling. "Heavy" soiling was more likely to occur in patients with a high/ intermediate malformation ("heavy"soiling: high/intermediate 10/16 vs low 2/17, p<0.01). It was also more common in males ("heavy" soiling: male 11/20 vs female 1/13, p<0.01) and patients who had undergone a PSARP ("heavy"soiling: PSARP 4/6, no PSARP 8/27, p<0.05).

Constipation (n=61) (Table 4)

We defined constipation as fewer than 3 stools per week or straining at stool for more than 25% of the time. Only 13% reported constipation occurring more than once a week. However, episodic constipation did occur. Twelve reported infrequent stools, 34 had hard stools and 39 had difficulty evacuating stools during the past year.

Patients with a low malformation were more likely to have had episodes of infrequent stooling during the past year (p<0.01).

Diarrhoea and rectal prolapse (n=57) (Table 5)

12% (7/57) of patients reported that episodes of diarrhoea occurred more than once a week. Patients with high/intermediate malformations were more likely to experience frequent episodes of diarrhoea.

Three patients (6% of 52) had constant anal excoriation and one had a rectal prolapse during the past year. Patients with a high/intermediate malformation were more likely to have perianal excoriation. Patients who had undergone a PSARP were also more likely to have perianal excoriation (excoriation: PSARP 3/8 vs no PSARP 6/44, p<0.05).

70% (42/60) of patients had episodic abdominal pain lasting more than two minutes. Of these, 10 reported abdominal pain 1 to 3 times per week and 9 reported pain 1 to 2 times per month. This was equally frequent in patients with a past history of either high/intermediate or low malformations.

		High/Intermediate n (%)	Low n (%)	p	Total n (%)
Constipation (n=61)	Never/Rarely/Sometimes	23 (85.2)	30(88.2)		53(86.9)
	Often/Always	4 (14.8)	4(11.8)	1.00	8(13.1)
Infrequent stool (in past year) n (%) (n=60)	Yes	1 (3.7)	11 (34.4)	0.00	12 (20.3)
If infrequent stools, number of episodes in last 3 months (n=9)		3.0 ± (-)	2.8±0.9	0.91	2.9±0.9
Hard stools (in past year) n (%)(n=60)	Yes	15 (53.6)	19 (59.4)	0.58	34 (56.7)
If hard stools, number of episodes in last 3 months (n=26)		5.5 ± 6.5	3.5 ± 3.3	0.35	4.5 ± 5.1
Difficulty in evacuating stool (in past year)	Yes	20 (71.4)	19 (59.4)	0.33	39 (65)
n (%) (n=60)					
If difficulty in evacuating stool, number of episodes in last 3 months (n=20)		7.0 ± 7.7	5.4 ± 7.1	0.63	6.1 ± 7.2

Table 4. Constipation data for interviewed patients.

Enuresis (n=56)

36% (20/56) of patients had enuresis at least once in the last 3 months. Nine had daytime enuresis, 8 had nocturnal enuresis and 3 had enuresis both during the day and at night. 16% of patients with daytime enuresis and 13% with night-time enuresis had an episode within the last week.

Patients with either daytime or nocturnal enuresis were younger than those who did not have enuresis (daytime enuresis 7.9 ± 5.0yr vs no enuresis 12.7 ± 6.3yr, $p<0.05$; nocturnal enuresis 9.0 ± 3.7yr vs no enuresis 13.1 ± 6.6yr, $p<0.05$).

		High/Intermediate n (%)	Low n (%)	p	Total n (%)
Diarrhoea (n=57)	Never/Rarely/Sometimes	20(76.9)	30(96.8)		50(87.7)
	Often / Always	6(23.1)	1(3.2)	0.04	7(12.3)
Excoriation (n=52)	Never	17(68)	26(96.3)		43(82.7)
	Sometimes	5(20)	1(3.7)		6(11.5)
	Always	3(12)	0(-)	0.02	3(5.8)
Rectal prolapse (n=59)	Yes	1(3.7)	0(-)	0.46	1(1.7)
Abdominal pain (n=60)	Yes	21(75)	21(65.6)	0.43	42(70)
Abdominal pain (frequency) (n=32)	1-6 times in past yr	6(37.4)	7(43.8)		13(40.6)
	1-2 times in past month	5(31.3)	4(25)		9(28.1)
	1-3 times in past wk	5(31.3)	5(31.2)	1.00	10(31.3)

Table 5. Diarrhoea data for interviewed patients.

Continence Aids (n=58)

29% (17/58) of patients used continence aids for soiling (6/17), enuresis (6/17) or both (5/17). Aids were used more frequently at night (12/58) than during the day (9/58). Daytime use was primarily for soiling, however nocturnal use was primarily for enuresis.

Patients with high/intermediate malformations were more likely to use aids at night (high/intermediate 8/26 vs low 4/32, $p<0.05$). Those who used aids overnight were younger than those who did not use them (continence aid use 7.7 ±3.6yr vs no use 12.7 ± 6.7yr, $p<0.05$).

Diet (n=61)

Over half (35/61) of patients reported adverse effects after some foods. Of these, 14 (40%) reported problems with fruit, 11 (31%) with vegetables, 16 (46%) with dairy, 12 (34%) with grains/breads/cereals, 13 (37%) with fatty or fast foods, 1 (3%) with meat, and 8 (23%) with other foods.

Overall, the most commonly reported adverse effects were diarrhoea (60%), constipation (28%) and abdominal discomfort (5%). Symptoms after fruit included diarrhoea (9/14, 64%), constipation (4/14, 29%) and peri-anal discomfort (2/14, 14%). Ingestion of vegetables was associated with diarrhoea (9/11, 82%) and constipation (1/11, 9%). Symptoms after dairy included diarrhoea (6/16, 38%), constipation (8/16, 50%) and abdominal discomfort (2/16, 13%). Grains/breads/cereals induced diarrhoea (7/12, 58%), constipation (3/12, 25%) and abdominal discomfort (1/12, 8%). Symptoms after fatty or fast foods included diarrhoea (7/13, 54%) and constipation (5/13, 38%). One patient experienced diarrhoea after meat.

54% (33/61) of patients either partially or totally restricted some foods from their diet because of these adverse effects. The most frequently restricted food groups were dairy (22%), fatty or fast foods (21%), fruit (17%) and vegetables (16%).

Medication (n=63)

Over half (34/62) of patients had used a medication or other treatment for bowel related problems in the past year. 29 patients used laxatives, 2 used anti-diarrhoeals and 10 used bowel washouts. Most (27/34) patients were using some form of treatment at the time of interview. Medication-users at the time of interview were significantly younger than those who did not use medication (current medication use 9.2 ± 4.7yr vs no medication 10.4 ± 5.3yr, $p<0.05$). Of those who were using medication, 12 were using more than one type of laxative. Those with a high/intermediate malformation were more likely to be using a medication (high/intermediate 20/28 vs low 14/34, $p<0.05$). Patients with soiling were also more likely to be using medication (soiling 27/44 vs no soiling 5/16, $p<0.05$). Those who used laxatives were significantly younger than those who used anti-diarrhoeals (mean age: laxative 8.9 ± 4.3yr vs anti-diarrhoeal 19.9 ± 2.4yr, $p<0.05$).

Physical and Social Aspects

6% (4/62) of patients had limited their physical activities because of soiling or odour.

Soiling interfered with social activities of 11 (19%) patients. Of these, 9 had some parental or self-imposed restrictions and 2 had extreme limitations. As expected, patients with soiling were more likely to have social limitations than patients without soiling (social limitation: soiling 11/40 vs no soiling 0/16, $p<0.05$). Odour from soiling was also responsible for interference with social activities in 14% (8/58) of patients. Of these, 5 patients were rarely affected and 3 were frequently affected.

When questioned on the level of dependency on toilet facilities, 3.5% (2/57) of patients had used toilet facilities at least once every 30 minutes, and 5% (3/57) had to use toilet facilities at least once every hour.

On average, patients had been absent from school 0.8 ± 2.4 days in the past two school terms.

Two of the 9 patients who were in part-time or full-time work reported some limitations to their employment because of bowel dysfunction.

Health Care (n=62)

58% (34/59) patients had not had a follow-up visit for their bowel in over a year. Of these, 15 had not had a follow-up visit in the past 5 years. Patients who had follow-up visits within the last year were younger (<1yr follow-up: young 0-11yr 20/39 vs old 12-33yr 5/20, $p<0.001$) and have a high/intermediate malformation ($p<0.05$). Patients with soiling were more likely to have had a follow-up visit in the past year (<1yr follow-up: soiling 19/41 vs no soiling 4/16, $p<0.05$).

12% (6/49) of patients who attended school had an integration aid for bowel related problems (ie. cleaning after soiling).

37% (23/62) of patients received financial assistance from the Commonwealth Government because of health issues (Health Care card). Patients with high/intermediate malformations

(Health Care card: high/intermediate 15/28 vs low 8/34, $p<0.05$) and patients with soiling were more likely to have a health care card (Health Care card: soiling 21/44 vs no soiling 2/16, $p<0.05$) for bowel related problems.

27% (17/62) of patients received financial assistance in the form of a Disability allowance or their families received Carer's allowances. Patients with soiling were more likely to have received Disability allowances (Disability allowance: soiling 16/54 vs no soiling 1/16, $p<0.05$) for bowel related problems.

Continence and Quality of Life Scores

Templeton continence scores could only be determined for 23% (14/62) of patients. Based on the Templeton classification, 3 patients had "poor", 6 "fair" and 5 had "good" continence.

The requirement for digital anal examination meant that Holschneider classification of continence was able only used in 23% of patients. Four were classified as having "fair" continence, 7 "good" and 3 "normal".

Classification of quality of life using the Ditesheim and Templeton scale was valid for 85% (53/62) of patients. Five patients had "fair" quality of life and 48 "good".

Manometry (n=12) (Table 6)

Baseline anal sphincter pressures were significantly less than normal reference ranges, but there was little difference between those who did and did not soil. Recto-anal inhibitory reflexes were present in 5 patients, but the threshold volume for eliciting the reflex was significantly greater than normal. Sensation to rectal distension was also blunted. Most were unable to evacuate a water filled rectal balloon normally.

Down's Syndrome Group (n=3)

The three patients with Down's syndrome and high/intermediate anorectal malformations were 12 ± 3.4 years old. Two were male and one female. Two had a redo PSARP operation. Co-morbidities included cardiac, gastrointestinal (non colorectal), renal and respiratory.

All three had a bowel action each day. Stool consistency was formed in two and pasty in one patient. Two patients could hold back stool more than 75% of the time.

All three had soiled within the past year. Three "often" had daytime soiling episodes. Daytime soiling varied between a pasty to formed consistency and streak to large amount. One "often" soiled nocturnally and two wore nappies at night.

Only one patient had constipation and abdominal pain. The other two had episodic diarrhoea, and one also had anal excoriation.

One patient had both day and night enuresis and one only had daytime enuresis in the last week.

One patient used incontinence aids day and night for enuresis and soiling and another also used incontinence aids for enuresis and soiling but only at night.

http://dx.doi.org/10.5772/57072

	Soiling Never//Sometimes	Soiling Often/Always	p	Total	Historical normal values	p
Baseline sphincter pressure (mean±SD)	38.1±20.8	37.9±20.8	0.99	38±19.4	53±12	<0.01
Recto-anal inhibitory reflex						
• Normal	1	1		2		
• Present but abnormal	1	2		3		
• Not present	1	4	0.64	5		
Recto-anal inhibitory reflex (if present) – threshold (mL)	35±7.1	32.5±15	0.84	33.3±12.1	16±7	<0.01
Sensation to distension (mL)	69±79.9	90±65.4	0.62	80.5±69.4	14±7	<0.01
Co-ordination						
• Relaxation	2	1		3		
• No change	2	2		4		
• Anismus	0	2	0.33	2	10%	
Ability to evacuate water-filled balloon						
100mL	1	1		2	100%	
50mL	1	2		3		
30mL	0	0		0		
Unable	2	4		6		

Table 6. Manometry results from 12 patients.

No patient had any limitations to their physical activities but one did limit social activities because of odour from soiling, and one needed access to toilet facilities every 30 minutes.

All patients had a health care card and received disability allowance.

Only two patients had a follow-up for their bowel in the past 12 months. One was using laxatives at the time of interview for bowel control and another patient had used laxatives in the past year but had ceased 4 months prior.

All three had adverse effects from foods. These foods included fruit, vegetables and fatty or fast foods. The effects from these foods included diarrhoea and abdominal discomfort.

Social impact of incontinence – parental free comments (overall group of 62)

Earlier diagnosis:

- One parent felt as though diagnosis (of ARM) could have been made sooner if they (parents) had been more assertive. It took a day to diagnose although the Mother knew that something was not right with her son after birth, despite the nurses saying that he was fine.

Genetics:

- Two mothers thought there might be a genetic link. One mother was concerned about her future pregnancies. Two mothers were also concerned about the chance of their children's children having malformations.

Social limitations:

- One patient was teased at school because she wore a nappy and this would really upset her. Two patients were limited in their social activities because they were embarrassed to sleep over at friends or did not go to camps because of inadequate toilet facilities. School was difficult for one boy because he had to go to the toilet quite frequently during class.

Coping:

- Parents and patients coped with the disease in various ways. Three parents said that you just have to deal with it, with one adding that that was her role as a mother. One family put the disease into perspective for their child by saying that it could be a lot worse. One parent felt that being open and not making a big deal would hopefully decrease the chance of problems in the future. One mother said that you "have to have a sense of humour or you just go nuts".
- One parent said that she had to block out how bad the anal dilatations were in order for her to perform them. Two patients said that they had learnt to deal with it, with one stating that there was no need to dwell on it and another saying that you would cope with whatever happened when it came. One mother said that at times her daughter was quite upset with her malformations and procedures, however she understands their need. One patient felt that there is nothing he can do so he just deals with it. One patient always asks his parents why it has happened to him. One patient used to ask why this happened to her and feel really helpless.
- One parent said that the disease affects the whole family, not just the patient. Three parents were quite distressed about having to give their children treatment (medication, bowel washouts or anal dilatations). One parent said that it was upsetting to see their child go through it all. One mother said that it was "mentally destroying" to hear her baby crying all the time when he was passing bowel actions. She said that she did not know how she coped without any help. One patient developed a fear of going to the toilet because he would be in so much pain.

Associated disabilities:

- There were some questions by both parents and patients surrounding physical ability and if this was the reason for soiling.

Medical interactions:

- A few parents wanted more follow-up visits to occur and at more frequent times so they could monitor their child's progress. One parent did not feel that there was a need to see her doctor because he did not offer her any new information.

4. Discussion

This review reaffirms the importance of problems with bowel control in the long term outcome after surgical repair of anorectal malformation. Over two thirds of patients had faecal incontinence over the past year and half of these had soiling which occurred either often or always. Half of all the patients soiled both during the day and at night. As expected, patients with high/intermediate malformations were more severely affected. The most severe "heavy" soiling occurred in approximately a fifth of the patients. These patients were more likely to be male or have high/intermediate malformations.

There was evidence that bowel control improved with age, but faecal urgency was still a problem in half of those aged 12 years and over. Children with low malformations tended to be less severely affected but there was also a suggestion of a slightly different symptom complex. Constipation was more common in patients with low malformation and diarrhoea more common in patients with high/intermediate malformations. Those with Down syndrome also had a poor outcome but we had no direct comparison group for this small number of children.

Only one quarter of potentially eligible patients in our study were surveyed. It is possible that this may have skewed the results toward a poorer outcome. Certainly, some studies do show rather better outcomes, with only 20% having faecal incontinence using some scoring systems [17]. However, other studies have shown broadly similar long term outcomes for continence and quality of life [18-21].

The long term functional impact in adults upon continence and quality of life can be devastating. Rintala et al. examined the outcome for adults (mean age 35 years) in terms of quality of life following surgical repair high or intermediate anomalies compared to low anomalies [22, 23]. This pair of controlled studies determined that good continence was present in only 18% of patients with high or intermediate anomalies and in 60% of those with low anomalies. Pelvic dysfunction extended into other areas. Sexual dysfunction was present in 30% of those with high or intermediate anomalies and 13% of those with low anomalies.

Further operations have been offered and there is some evidence supporting a role for posterior sagittal anorectoplasty (PSARP) with or without provision of an antegrade continent enema in selected patients with persistent and unresponsive soiling [24]. However, in our study, soiling persisted even in those patients who had received a PSARP, suggesting that it may improve function it does not usually return bowel function to normal.

Other therapies have been offered. Biofeedback has been suggested in uncontrolled studies to provide substantial improvement in continence after surgical repair of ARM [25-28]. This should be evaluated critically as biofeedback has shown similar promise in uncontrolled studies of childhood encopresis which disappeared when evaluated within the framework of fully case-controlled trials [29].

Enuresis was also a problem in many patients. Some of these children may have also had urinary system anomalies. Where they occur, it has been suggested that they are at least as serious and complex as gastrointestinal anomalies, and contribute substantially to long term morbidity [17].

The social impacts of chronic gastrointestinal and urinary dysfunction are substantial. Approximately a quarter of the respondents in our study were on some form of financial health care assistance. Some of the comments made by parents would seem to go against the relatively optimistic outcomes on quality of life as determined by the Ditesheim and Templeton scale in our study, which suggested over three-quarters had a "good" quality of life. Quality of life measures can be extremely difficult to establish and there may be a case for looking more carefully at developing more specific and sensitive parameters [10].

An interesting observation was the impact of diet on bowel dysfunction. There is relatively little information on this area in the literature although an earlier study by the same authors in children with Hirschsprung disease identified similar findings in that group [14]. Many of the food groups which were problematic included either fibre-containing products (vegetables), lactose (dairy) or grains. There has certainly been a great deal of recent interest in the impact of rapidly fermentable, short-chain carbohydrates on functional bowel disease [30]. These have been given the acronym "FODMAPS", and found to have a substantial impact on functional abdominal pain, bloating and diarrhoea which are symptoms of irritable bowel syndrome [30]. Why this should be a particular problem in children after anorectal surgery such as Hirschsprung or anorectal malformation is not clear but may relate to the loss of a "rectal brake".

The assessment of residual function can be difficult. Several clinical-based protocols have been developed, but are poorly standardized with poor inter-scale correlation [31]. Anorectal manometry can identify a range of dysfunctional parameters which might be thought likely to contribute to incontinence [32]. In our study, a number of indices were markedly abnormal. Sphincter pressures were low. Sensory thresholds to rectal distension were extremely blunted. The rectoanal inhibitory reflex was often impaired, or only elicited with very high rectal distending volumes. Incoordinate defaecation was common, as was inability to evacuate a water filled balloon. What is interesting is that there was very little statistical difference between those who soiled heavily and those who had little soiling in terms of anorectal manometric parameters. It is likely that other pathophysiological "triggers" tip the balance in favour of heavy soiling.

Rapid colonic transit may be one such trigger. Ingestion of rapidly fermentable, short-chain carbohydrates is quite likely to lead to more rapid movement of luminal content with the potential for overcoming rectal control. There are varying abilities to tolerate fermentable loads, and these depend (amongst other factors) on rate of ingestion, concomitant nutrients, small intestinal processing, and colonic flora together with their metabolic activities. There is substantially more diversity in colonic flora than previously thought, with close interactions between environment, host genotype and the metabolic functioning gut microbiome [33]. If gut microbiome does play a role in faecal incontinence in this group, however minor, it represents an opportunity for therapeutic intervention.

http://dx.doi.org/10.5772/57072

Author details

Anthony G. Catto-Smith[1,3*], Misel Trajanovska[1,4] and Russell Taylor[2]

*Address all correspondence to: tony.cattosmith@rch.org.au

1 Dept of Gastroenterology and Clinical Nutrition, Royal Children's Hospital, Australia

2 Dept of Surgery, Royal Children's Hospital, Australia

3 Dept of Paediatrics, University of Melbourne, Australia

4 Murdoch Childrens Research Institute, Melbourne, Australia

References

[1] Cho S, Moore SP, Fangman T. One Hundred Three Consecutive Patients With Anorectal Malformations and Their Associated Anomalies. Arch Pediatr Adolesc Med. 2001 5/2001;155(5):587-91.

[2] Shaul DB, Harrison EA. Classification of anorectal malformations--initial approach, diagnostic tests, and colostomy. Semin Pediatr Surg. 1997 11/1997;6(4):187-95.

[3] Ong NT, Beasley SW. Long-term continence in patients with high and intermediate anorectal anomalies treated by sacroperineal (Stephens) rectoplasty. J Pediatr Surg. 1991 1/1991;26(1):44-8.

[4] Langemeijer RA, Molenaar JC. Continence after posterior sagittal anorectoplasty. J Pediatr Surg. 1991 5/1991;26(5):587-90.

[5] Templeton JM, Jr., Ditesheim JA. High imperforate anus--quantitative results of long-term fecal continence. J Pediatr Surg. 1985 12/1985;20(6):645-52.

[6] Holschneider AM, Pfrommer W, Gerresheim B. Results in the treatment of anorectal malformations with special regard to the histology of the rectal pouch. Eur J Pediatr Surg. 1994 Oct;4(5):303-9.

[7] Kelly JH. The clinical and radiological assessment of anal continence in childhood. Aust N Z J Surg. 1972 8/1972;42(1):62-3.

[8] Kiesewetter WB, Chang JH. Imperforate Anus: a five to thirty year follow-up perspective. ProgPediatrSurg. 1977 1977;10:111-20.

[9] Stephens FD, Durham-Smith E. Classification, identification, and assessment of surgical treatment of anorectal anomalies. Pediatr Surg Int. 1986 1986;1:200-5.

[10] Trajanovska M, Catto-Smith AG. Quality of life measures for fecal incontinence and their use in children. J Gastroenterol Hepatol. 2005 Jun;20(6):919-28.

[11] Stephens FD, Smith ED. Classification. In: Stephens FD, Smith ED, editors. Anorectal malformations in children. Chicago: Year Book Medical Publishers; 1971.

[12] Catto-Smith AG, Coffey CM, Nolan TM, Hutson JM. Fecal incontinence after the surgical treatment of Hirschsprung disease. J Pediatr. 1995 12/1995;127(6):954-7.

[13] Catto-Smith AG, Trajanovska M, Taylor RG. Long-term continence in patients with Hirschsprung's disease and Down syndrome. J Gastroenterol Hepatol. 2006 Apr; 21(4):748-53.

[14] Catto-Smith A, Trajanovska M, Taylor R. Long term continence after surgery for Hirschsprung's disease. J Gastroenterol Hepatol. 2007;22(12):2273-82.

[15] Catto-Smith AG, Nolan TM, Coffey CM. Clinical significance of anismus in encopresis. J Gastroenterol Hepatol. 1998 9/1998;13(9):955-60.

[16] Dewan PA, Elsworthy E, Mathew M, Poki O, Khaw SL, Roberts K, et al. Bowel imbrication in the management of anorectal anomalies. Pediatr Surg Int. 2004 Sep;20(9): 708-13.

[17] Senel E, Akbiyik F, Atayurt H, Tiryaki HT. Urological problems or fecal continence during long-term follow-up of patients with anorectal malformation. Pediatr Surg Int. 2010 Jul;26(7):683-9.

[18] Schmidt D, Jenetzky E, Zwink N, Schmiedeke E, Maerzheuser S. Postoperative complications in adults with anorectal malformation: a need for transition. German Network for Congenital Uro-REctal Malformations (CURE-Net). Pediatr Surg Int. 2012 Aug;28(8):793-5.

[19] Pruthi GK, Mohta A. Psychosocial burden and quality of life in parents of children with anorectal malformation. J Indian Assoc Pediatr Surg. 2010 Jan;15(1):15-8.

[20] Bai Y, Yuan Z, Wang W, Zhao Y, Wang H, Wang W. Quality of life for children with fecal incontinence after surgically corrected anorectal malformation. J Pediatr Surg. 2000 3/2000;35(3):462-4.

[21] Stenstrom P, Kockum CC, Bener DK, Ivarsson C, Arnbjornsson E. Adolescents with anorectal malformation: physical outcome, sexual health and quality of life. Int J Adolesc Med Health. 2013 May 1:1-11.

[22] Rintala R, Mildh L, Lindahl H. Fecal continence and quality of life in adult patients with an operated low anorectal malformation. J Pediatr Surg. 1992 7/1992;27(7):902-5.

[23] Rintala R, Mildh L, Lindahl H. Fecal continence and quality of life for adult patients with an operated high or intermediate anorectal malformation. J Pediatr Surg. 1994 6/1994;29(6):777-80.

[24] Ardelean MA, Bauer J, Schimke C, Ludwikowski B, Schimpl G. Improvement of continence with reoperation in selected patients after surgery for anorectal malformation. Dis Colon Rectum. 2009 Jan;52(1):112-8.

[25] Martins JL, Pinus J. Use of biofeedback (BFB) in the treatment of fecal incontinence after surgical correction of anorectal malformations by posterior sagittal anorectoplasty (PSARP). Sao Paulo Med J. 1997 5/1997;115(3):1427-32.

[26] Iwai N, Iwata G, Kimura O, Yanagihara J. Is a new biofeedback therapy effective for fecal incontinence in patients who have anorectal malformations? J Pediatr Surg. 1997 11/1997;32(11):1626-9.

[27] Rintala R, Lindahl H, Louhimo I. Biofeedback conditioning for fecal incontinence in anorectal malformations. Pediatr Surg Int. 1988 1988;3:418-21.

[28] Leung MW, Wong BP, Leung AK, Cho JS, Leung ET, Chao NS, et al. Electrical stimulation and biofeedback exercise of pelvic floor muscle for children with faecal incontinence after surgery for anorectal malformation. Pediatr Surg Int. 2006 Dec;22(12): 975-8.

[29] Loening-Baucke V. Biofeedback training in children with functional constipation. A critical review. Dig Dis Sci. 1996 Jan;41(1):65-71.

[30] Gibson PR, Shepherd SJ. Evidence-based dietary management of functional gastrointestinal symptoms: The FODMAP approach. J Gastroenterol Hepatol. 2010 Feb;25(2): 252-8.

[31] Ochi T, Okazaki T, Miyano G, Lane GJ, Yamataka A. A comparison of clinical protocols for assessing postoperative fecal continence in anorectal malformation. Pediatr Surg Int. 2011 Jan;28(1):1-4.

[32] Senel E, Demirbag S, Tiryaki T, Erdogan D, Cetinkursun S, Cakmak O. Postoperative anorectal manometric evaluation of patients with anorectal malformation. Pediatr Int. 2007 Apr;49(2):210-4.

[33] Spor A, Koren O, Ley R. Unravelling the effects of the environment and host genotype on the gut microbiome. Nat Rev Microbiol. 2011 Apr;9(4):279-90.